T0255730

ORTHOPEDIC
Residency & Fellowship

A GUIDE TO SUCCESS

ORTHOPEDIC
Residency & Fellowship

A GUIDE TO SUCCESS

Laith M. Jazrawi, MD
Assistant Professor, NYU School of Medicine
Chief, Sports Medicine Division
Director, Surgical Skills Lab
Director of Sports and Shoulder/Elbow Research Lab
NYU Hospital for Joint Diseases
Department of Orthopaedic Surgery
New York University
New York, NY

Kenneth A. Egol, MD
Associate Professor and Vice Chairman
NYU Hospital for Joint Diseases
Department of Orthopaedic Surgery
New York University
New York, NY

Joseph D. Zuckerman, MD
Professor and Chairman
NYU Hospital for Joint Diseases
Department of Orthopaedic Surgery
New York University
New York, NY

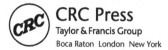

CRC Press
Taylor & Francis Group
Boca Raton London New York

CRC Press is an imprint of the
Taylor & Francis Group, an **informa** business

This book has been published in a previous form by NYU Hospital for Joint Diseases Department of Orthopaedic Surgery as *Orthopaedic Residency: How to Get Into a Program and Succeed Once You're There.*

First published 2010 by SLACK Incorporated

Published 2024 by CRC Press
2385 NW Executive Center Drive, Suite 320, Boca Raton FL 33431

and by CRC Press
4 Park Square, Milton Park, Abingdon, Oxon, OX14 4RN

CRC Press is an imprint of Taylor & Francis Group, LLC

© 2010 Taylor & Francis Group, LLC

This book contains information obtained from authentic and highly regarded sources. While all reasonable efforts have been made to publish reliable data and information, neither the author[s] nor the publisher can accept any legal responsibility or liability for any errors or omissions that may be made. The publishers wish to make clear that any views or opinions expressed in this book by individual editors, authors or contributors are personal to them and do not necessarily reflect the views/opinions of the publishers. The information or guidance contained in this book is intended for use by medical, scientific or health-care professionals and is provided strictly as a supplement to the medical or other professional's own judgement, their knowledge of the patient's medical history, relevant manufacturer's instructions and the appropriate best practice guidelines. Because of the rapid advances in medical science, any information or advice on dosages, procedures or diagnoses should be independently verified. The reader is strongly urged to consult the relevant national drug formulary and the drug companies' and device or material manufacturers' printed instructions, and their websites, before administering or utilizing any of the drugs, devices or materials mentioned in this book. This book does not indicate whether a particular treatment is appropriate or suitable for a particular individual. Ultimately it is the sole responsibility of the medical professional to make his or her own professional judgements, so as to advise and treat patients appropriately. The authors and publishers have also attempted to trace the copyright holders of all material reproduced in this publication and apologize to copyright holders if permission to publish in this form has not been obtained. If any copyright material has not been acknowledged please write and let us know so we may rectify in any future reprint.

Except as permitted under U.S. Copyright Law, no part of this book may be reprinted, reproduced, transmitted, or utilized in any form by any electronic, mechanical, or other means, now known or hereafter invented, including photocopying, microfilming, and recording, or in any information storage or retrieval system, without written permission from the publishers.

For permission to photocopy or use material electronically from this work, access www.copyright.com or contact the Copyright Clearance Center, Inc. (CCC), 222 Rosewood Drive, Danvers, MA 01923, 978-750-8400. For works that are not available on CCC please contact mpkbookspermissions@tandf.co.uk

Trademark notice: Product or corporate names may be trademarks or registered trademarks and are used only for identification and explanation without intent to infringe.

Library of Congress Cataloging-in-Publication Data

Orthopedic residency & fellowship : a guide to success / [edited by] Laith M. Jazrawi, Kenneth A. Egol, Joseph D. Zuckerman.
      p. ; cm.
   Includes bibliographical references and index.
   ISBN 9781556429309 (alk. paper)
   1. Orthopedics--Study and teaching (Residency)--United States. I. Jazrawi, Laith M., 1969- II. Egol, Kenneth A., 1967- III. Zuckerman, Joseph D. (Joseph David), 1952- IV. Title: Orthopedic residency and fellowship.
   [DNLM: 1. Internship and Residency. 2. Orthopedics--education. 3. Schools, Medical. 4. Vocational Guidance. WE 18 O767 2010]
   RD732.O78 2010
   616.7'023--dc22
                              2009050481

ISBN: 9781556429309 (pbk)
ISBN: 9781003525486 (ebk)

DOI: 10.1201/9781003525486

DEDICATION

To my beautiful and supportive wife, Adela, and daughters, Taylor, Isabella, and Victoria. Thank you for your unconditional love and support.
Laith M. Jazrawi, MD

To the residents and students at the NYU Hospital for Joint Diseases who make going to work every day enjoyable, and to my wife, Lori, and children, Alex, Jonathan, and Gabby, who make coming home even better.
Kenneth A. Egol, MD

To my wife, Janet, and my sons, Scott and Matthew—the joys of my life.
Joseph D. Zuckerman, MD

CONTENTS

Section I

Section II

Contents

Section III

Appendices

ACKNOWLEDGMENTS

In conversation after conversation in which medical students sought our advice on how to pursue an orthopedic residency, the authors were struck by how little information on this subject was available in print. We also realized that there is a similar lack of material on how to survive and succeed during the rigors of orthopedic residency training. Looking back on our own experiences, it was evident that most of this information was obtained from the residents ahead of us—those with somewhat more experience who "had been there." Although it was all extremely useful, it was, in many ways, incomplete. Fulfilling the need for a comprehensive text on strategies to successfully match to an orthopedic residency program and how to succeed once you are there was the driving force behind the first edition. The very positive feedback we received on the first edition and its extensive use throughout the country were the driving forces behind our decision to complete this second edition.

We are grateful to the many individuals who used the first edition and provided us with suggestions for the second edition. We would especially like to recognize the contributions of Lava Patel and Michael Day for their assistance in preparing the second edition. We would also like to thank the faculty, staff, and residents at NYU Hospital for Joint Diseases for their input and support. We recognize that the subject matter of this book is constantly changing and we have made every effort to be as current as possible. In that context, it is always a good idea to check the sources of the material included for any updates.

Orthopedic residency training remains one of the most competitive specialties. We hope this book serves you well in medical school, during the application process, and throughout your residency. To each and every reader of the textbook, we wish you success in all of your future pursuits.

ABOUT THE EDITORS

Laith M. Jazrawi, MD is an associate professor of orthopedics at the New York University (NYU) Langone Medical Center and Chief of the Sports Medicine Division. He also serves as Director of the Surgical Skills Lab and Sports & Shoulder/Elbow Research Laboratory.

Kenneth A. Egol, MD is a professor of orthopedic surgery at NYU School of Medicine, Chief of the Trauma Division at NYU Hospital for Joint Diseases, and Vice Chairman for the Department of Orthopaedic Surgery at NYU Hospital for Joint Diseases. He is Director of the NYU Hospital for Joint Diseases Orthopaedic Residency Program that currently trains 62 residents.

Joseph D. Zuckerman, MD is the Walter A. L. Thompson Professor of orthopedic surgery at the NYU School of Medicine and Chairman of the Department of Orthopaedic Surgery at NYU Hospital for Joint Diseases. He served as Director of the Orthopaedic Surgery Residency Program at the NYU Hospital for Joint Diseases from 1990-1997 and the combined NYU Hospital for Joint Diseases Program from 1997-2006.

Contributing Authors

Andrew E. Blustein, Esq (Chapter 19)
Attorney at Law
Partner-Director
Garfunkel Wild, P.C.

Kirk A. Campbell, MD (Chapter 10)
Orthopedic Resident
Hospital for Joint Diseases
Department of Orthopaedic Surgery
New York University
New York, NY

Craig J. Della Valle, MD (Chapter 17)
Associate Professor, Orthopedic Surgery
Rush University Medical Center
Chicago, IL

Lawrence B. Keller, CFP®, CLU, ChFC,
  RHU, LUTCF (Chapter 16)
Certified Financial Planner™ professional
Physician Financial Services
Woodbury, NY

Suezie Kim, MD (Chapter 13)
Orthopedic Surgery Resident
Hospital for Joint Diseases
Department of Orthopaedic Surgery
New York University
New York, NY

Catherine Laible, MD (Chapter 13)
Orthopedic Resident
Hospital for Joint Diseases
Department of Orthopaedic Surgery
NYU Langone Medical Center
New York, NY

Steve K. Lee, MD (Chapter 17)
Assistant Professor, NYU School of
  Medicine
Associate Chief, Division of Hand Surgery
Hospital for Joint Diseases
Department of Orthopaedic Surgery
New York University
Co-Chief, Hand Surgery Service
Bellevue Hospital Center
New York, NY

Daniel M. Lerman, MD (Chapter 7)
Orthopedic Resident
Hospital for Joint Diseases
Department of Orthopaedic Surgery
New York University
New York, NY

Crispin C. Ong, MD (Chapter 4)
Orthopedic Surgery Resident
Hospital for Joint Diseases
Department of Orthopaedic Surgery
New York University
New York, NY

Lava Y. Patel, BA (Chapters 2, 3, 8, & 17)
Research Coordinator
Hospital for Joint Diseases
Department of Orthopaedic Surgery
New York University
New York, NY

Carl Paulino, MD (Chapter 8)
Associate Program Director
Assistant Clinical Professor, Orthopedic
  Surgery
SUNY Downstate Medical Center
Brooklyn, NY

Afshin Eli Razi, MD (Chapter 17)
Clinical Assistant Professor, Orthopedic
  Surgery
Hospital for Joint Diseases
Department of Orthopaedic Surgery
New York University
New York, NY

David E. Ruchelsman, MD (Chapters 2, 4,
  7, 11, 14, & 15)
Fellow, Hand, Upper Extremity, and
  Microvascular Surgery Service
Department of Orthopaedic Surgery
Massachusetts General Hospital
Harvard Medical School
Boston, MA

Eric J. Strauss, MD (Chapters 3, 10, 11, 14, & 15)
Assistant Professor
Hospital For Joint Diseases
Department of Orthopaedic Surgery
Division of Sports Medicine
New York University
New York, NY

Brett Young, MD (Chapter 17)
Shoulder and Elbow Fellow
Hospital for Joint Diseases
New York University
New York, NY

PREFACE

Orthopedic surgery is a wonderful specialty. Its attractiveness is evident in the large number of applicants that apply for orthopedic residency positions each year. For many years, the number of applicants has far exceeded the number of available post-graduate year 1 (PGY-1) positions; this is true even when only considering the number of applicants applying from US medical schools.

There is no single factor that will ensure that an applicant will successfully match to an orthopedic surgery residency program. Rather, it is a combination of factors that make an applicant attractive to residency programs, including academic, experiential, and interpersonal attributes. Our purpose in preparing this text is to provide medical students with information that will increase their chances of successfully matching to an orthopedic residency program and, once there, to provide guidance about how to be successful during residency training, including obtaining fellowship training.

At NYU Hospital for Joint Diseases, we have had extensive experience in residency training. One of us (Dr. Zuckerman) served as Program Director from 1990 to 2006. In 1998, we combined the residency programs of the Hospital for Joint Diseases (with 6 residents per year) and NYU Medical Center (6 residents per year) into a program that now trains 12 residents each year. We have had experience with medical students from all over the country rotating at our institutions. The first edition of this textbook, published in 2003, was the concept of Dr. Jazrawi when he was still a resident. It was prepared by members of our faculty and members of our residency program to provide the faculty perspective on specific topics and the resident perspective on others. We were very careful to match the topic with the contributor in order to provide the most useful information. We could not have predicted the success of the first edition. Even though we published the book ourselves and primarily distributed it to medical students who visited our institution, we required multiple printings to fulfill the demand. This was the reason we decided to proceed with a second edition.

The information included in this book will be very helpful to any medical student who would like to pursue residency training in orthopedic surgery. The earlier it is used during medical school, the more helpful it will be. It will also be helpful for anyone beginning his or her orthopedic residency training by providing a strategy for success—not only during residency but after residency as well. At NYU Hospital for Joint Diseases, we are very, very proud of our commitment to orthopedic education at all levels, from the undergraduate level to medical school to orthopedic residency and fellowship training to CME for practicing orthopedic surgeons. This book—*Orthopedic Residency & Fellowship: A Guide to Success*—is another example of our commitment.

Laith M. Jazrawi, MD
Kenneth A. Egol, MD
Joseph D. Zuckerman, MD

Section I

EVALUATION OF THE APPLICANT

THE PROGRAM DIRECTOR'S PERSPECTIVE

With all of the constraints facing medical education programs today, such as work hour restrictions, a changing economy and its accompanying financial pressures, and the current generation of physicians' emphasis on a balanced lifestyle, it is imperative for orthopedic educators to identify and select the best possible residents to fill our residency programs. These issues have been addressed in several recent editorials from major orthopedic journals with specific emphasis placed on identifying medical student qualities that maximize the chances of success during residency. One such commentary stressed that continuously refining and improving resident education and training are of the utmost importance to the future of orthopedic surgery today because doing so will facilitate the continued recruitment of top medical students.[1]

Orthopedic surgery has been and continues to be among the most competitive fields in postgraduate medical training. Nearly 100% of first post-graduate year (PGY-1) residency spots in orthopedics are filled yearly, and the majority of these are filled by American medical school graduates.[2-4] In 2008, there were 160 orthopedic surgery residency programs that participated in the National Resident Matching Program (NRMP). These programs offered a total of 636 positions, of which 99.8% were filled (93.1% with US medical students).[5]

That year was similar to previous years in which the overwhelming majority of applicants matching have been US allopathic medical students. In 2008, only one program was left unfilled. There were 932 applicants (740 from the US) for the 636 available positions. Of the 635 matched spots, 592 (93.1%) were filled by US senior medical students. In 2008, the relative ratio of residency positions to applicants was 0.7. For 683 of the 740 applicants from US allopathic medical schools, orthopedic surgery was their only residency choice; for 48 it was their first but not only choice; and for 9 applicants it was second to another subspecialty. So, for those US medical students who only applied to orthopedic surgery for residency, there was a 16% unmatched rate. For "independent applicants" (eg, osteopaths, international medical graduates), more than 74% did not match. Additional analysis of the NRMP data indicates that, on average, residency programs need to rank 5 applicants for each available orthopedic position.[5]

Kenneth A. Egol, MD

L. M. Jazrawi, K. A. Egol, & J. D. Zuckerman.
Orthopedic Residency & Fellowship: A Guide to Success (pp. 3-8)
© 2010 Taylor & Francis Group.

The specific academic criteria or personal attributes that programs use to assess potential candidates varies somewhat, but in general, students accepted into orthopedic residencies are generally at the top of their medical school classes, perform well on the United States Medical Licensing Examination (USMLE) Step 1, are involved in some type of research activity, and perform a number of visiting orthopedic elective rotations. Medical students who match into orthopedic surgery are of high academic caliber.

MEDICAL SCHOOL GRADES/USMLE STEP 1

Different medical schools use a variety of grading options. Most are pass/fail, honors/pass/fail, or honors/high pass/pass/fail. We tend to assess academic excellence by the number of honors grades obtained. More weight is given to grades of honors in the clinical years compared with the pre-clinical years. For schools without honors grades, the USMLE may be the only way to distinguish these students amongst their peers. The median USMLE Step 1 score is 230 for those obtaining an orthopedic residency spot—the third highest among all specialties (behind plastic surgery and dermatology).

MEDICAL STUDENT HONOR SOCIETY

Selection for Alpha Omega Alpha (AΩA) is usually associated with being in the top 10% to 15% of a medical student's class. Different medical schools use different criteria for selection, but the consistent theme is the highest level of academic achievement. Some medical schools do not have a chapter of AΩA, and applicants are able to identify this fact on their Electronic Residency Application Service (ERAS) applications. While not a prerequisite for gaining an interview at our program, up to two-thirds of those granted an interview are members of AΩA.

RESEARCH ACTIVITY

Almost all of the applicants we interview have participated in some type of research. The degree and level of participation varies. Most students applying for orthopedic surgery will have been involved in a defined clinical research investigation. Some will have dedicated a full year or more to scientific pursuits. Finally, the rare candidate will have completed an MD/PhD program with a significant amount of time dedicated to basic science research. These activities, in concert with the applicant's academic record, help to identify the strongest candidates. There are several points to consider when beginning a pursuit of research. First, no amount of research can make up for a poor academic record. Potential candidates should consider whether time to be spent on a research project might be better spent studying for a medical school core course or the USMLE. Consider using electives or summers off for research activity. Second, quality trumps quantity. I would rather see an applicant with one good quality project to which he or she made a significant contribution to and saw through to publication than someone who has his or her name on a number of abstracts that he or she "tagged along on" and had little involvement with. When interviewing, the applicant should have an in-depth knowledge of his or her research and be able to discuss it in detail. Inability to do so is a red flag to interviewers about the accuracy of the application. Overall, nearly two-thirds of orthopedic applicants have authored publications, and 9 out of 10 have participated in research activities.[6]

AWAY ROTATIONS

A recent survey of program directors identified the "clinical orthopedic elective" at the director's institution as a major determinant of selection into an orthopedic residency program. Approximately half of the applicants we interview have performed a clerkship with us. These rotations give the applicant the chance to learn about our program, and it gives us the chance to get to know the applicant to a much greater degree than from a relatively short day of interviews. Personal attributes such as work ethic, interpersonal skills, and dedication become apparent and greatly increase the applicant's chances of matching at a particular institution if the rotation has been a successful one. An away rotation does not always guarantee an interview. It is important to keep in mind that a less-than-stellar performance during an "on-site" rotation will significantly weaken what otherwise might have been a very strong "paper" application.

LETTERS OF RECOMMENDATION

These letters of recommendation are an important aspect of the application. Each student must obtain a letter from his or her dean of students. These letters are lengthy and encompass the entire academic record of the candidate. At the end of the dean's letter, there is often a statement about the applicant, indicating his or her "standing" or "rank" amongst classmates. These letters provide very valuable information, with some schools indicating that the highest descriptor applies to the top 10% of students, and others the top 30%. Frequently, the second-level standing applies to the next 40% to 50% of the class, thereby making differentiation of candidates from one another difficult. Outside of the dean's letter, most programs require at least 3 letters of recommendation from faculty or physicians who know the applicant very well. Most programs require one of these letters to be from the chairman of the orthopedic department at your medical school, so check the requirements of each program you apply to. When choosing someone to write a letter of recommendation for you, choose someone who will be able to illustrate those personal attributes that will make you stand out among your peers. This faculty member need not be an orthopedic surgeon. A very strong letter from a non-orthopedist is preferable to a mediocre letter from an orthopedic faculty member.

PERSONAL STATEMENT

The personal statement provides the applicant the chance to call attention to specific aspects of his or her academic record or outside achievements that may strengthen the application. Certain life experiences, additional skills, and qualifications will help convey to the reader that he or she has more to offer and possesses a level of maturity or significant drive to succeed, which will make him or her a more attractive candidate to the reviewers. With that said, the personal statement has less impact on my review of the application than the other components. The majority of statements are similar, with most applicants tracing their interest in the field to some remote orthopedic injury or sporting accident with a personal journey through recovery that has shaped their desire. In general, it is better to follow the standard formula rather than try to "stand out" with a statement that emphasizes creativity over substance.

OUTSIDE ACTIVITIES

I believe that outside extracurricular activities are important and give me a sense about the "whole person." Activities such as involvement in undergraduate athletics (especially in leadership roles); musical involvement; work with charitable organizations; and accomplishments in fields other than medicine, writing, or military service all indicate well-rounded individuals who have a track record of success and the ability to work well with others (team player). These are attributes I find extremely important, and, as such, I have placed considerably more weight on these attributes in recent years.

Currently and for the past 20 years, resident selection decisions have been made by a committee of faculty at our institution that reviews all of the applications and then generates a consensus ranking of all of the applicants to determine those to be granted an interview. The number of applicants is typically large (between 400 and 500 including foreign applicants), and the means by which such decisions are made is subjective and specific to our individual program. While we try to evaluate the candidate as a whole, we use certain criteria to identify the pool of applicants who will be evaluated further, by means of a formal interview.

We have recently identified several of these pre-residency criteria that predicted a successful performance in our orthopedic surgery residency program. We evaluated 150 residents who matched into our university-based residency program over a 20-year period. Our results indicated that purely academic pre-residency selection factors, including medical school rank and USMLE Step 1 score, are positively correlated with higher average percentile scores on the Orthopaedic In-Training Exam (OITE). Because students at higher ranked medical schools often have performed better on standardized testing (higher MCAT scores), it is logical that these students, as well as those who scored highest on USMLE Step 1, would be most likely to succeed in another standardized testing environment such as the OITE. However, other non-academic pre-selection factors that correlated with success in a training program include completing a rotation at our institution where the faculty could get to know the applicant to a greater degree and a history of significant involvement in charitable activities. Interestingly, we did not find a positive correlation between any predictor and passing the American Board of Orthopaedic Surgery (ABOS) examination on the first attempt. This may have been due to the very high number of residents who successfully completed Part I on the first try (142/147, or 97%).

While it is clear that there is no one specific path into an orthopedic residency program, candidates possess several common character traits. Successful orthopedic candidates are highly motivated individuals with a strong moral character. These students are highly intelligent and well-rounded. Clearly, these individuals are driven and determined. According to the NRMP, applicants are more likely to be successful if they rank several programs in their desired specialty. Medical students who were successfully matched into orthopedic surgery residencies in 2008 ranked about 11 orthopedic programs.[7]

Finally, we support the goals of the American Academy of Orthopaedic Surgeons (AAOS) in fostering diversity in orthopedics by supporting efforts to diversify the profession and orthopedic workforce. As part of these efforts, our training program is committed to identifying and training qualified women and under-represented minorities who are interested in the field of orthopedic surgery.

REFERENCES

1. Lehman WB. Educating our residents: more important than ever. *Am J Orthop*. 2007;36(12): E171, E189.

2. Signer MM, Beran RL. Results of the National Resident Matching Program for 2003. *Acad Med*. 2003;78(6):653-656.

3. Signer MM, Beran RL. Results of the National Resident Matching Program for 2004. *Acad Med*. 2004;79(6):610-612.

4. Signer MM, Beran RL. Results of the National Resident Matching Program for 2005. *Acad Med*. 2005;80(6):610-612.

5. National Resident Matching Program. *Advanced Data Tables: 2008 Main Residency Match*. 2008. Available at: http://www.nrmp.org/data/advancedatatables2008.pdf. Accessed November 17, 2009.

6. National Resident Matching Program. *Charting Outcomes in the Match: Characteristics of Applicants Who Matched to Their Preferred Specialty in the 2009 NRMP Main Residency Match*. 3rd ed. 2009. Available at: http://www.nrmp.org/data/chartingoutcomes2009v3. pdf. Accessed November 17, 2009.

7. Chapralis S. Resident education: striking the right match. 2008. Available at: http://www. aaos.org/news/bulletin/may07/research3.asp. Accessed November 17, 2009.

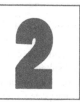

MEDICAL SCHOOL: THE EARLY YEARS

During the early years of medical school, the majority of matriculating students will not yet have determined or even considered the field in which they will pursue their career. For most, the clinical years of medical school will be the time when the scope of each major specialty will be discovered.

For the student who believes early on that orthopedic surgery is a serious potential career consideration, there are several ways to gain initial exposure to the specialty and its many subspecialties. These exposures and "connections" have the potential to become invaluable during the clinical years of medical school, the "match" process, and beyond.

This chapter elucidates several avenues through which the pre-clinical medical student may gain exposure to the field of orthopedic surgery, his or her institution's faculty members, and its resident physicians. It is through these early exposures and experiences that one may determine if a career in orthopedics is right.

PRIORITY NUMBER 1: ACADEMIC EXCELLENCE IN THE PRE-CLINICAL CURRICULUM

During the first 2 years of medical school, the primary focus should always be on academic responsibilities. Academic excellence in all coursework during the pre-clinical (first 2 years) curriculum is an essential component of a successful residency application. Superior academic achievement in these years represents the obtainment of a solid foundation upon which you will build your clinical knowledge, and it truly prepares you to excel on the United States Medical Licensing Examination (USMLE) Step 1 examination and on the wards as a clinical clerk. Outstanding scores during these 2 formidable years are the cornerstone on which you will be viewed as a competitive applicant to any specialty when you apply for residency positions. Some medical schools award junior Alpha Omega Alpha (AΩA) status based on academic achievement in the pre-clinical years, and this should be the goal of each student who wishes to pursue a career in orthopedic surgery.

Lava Y. Patel, BA and David E. Ruchelsman, MD

L. M. Jazrawi, K. A. Egol, & J. D. Zuckerman.
Orthopedic Residency & Fellowship: A Guide to Success (pp. 9-14)
© 2010 Taylor & Francis Group.

It should be stressed that performance of clinical and/or basic science research, completion of sub-internships, strong letters of recommendation, and participation in extracurricular activities only supplement and strengthen your residency application; these cannot fully compensate for a suboptimal academic performance during the pre-clinical years. Your grades are a top consideration for many program directors; however, there is more stress on clinical grades (see Chapter 1). In 2002, for example, 70% of program directors who were surveyed and asked to rank 26 different selection criteria ranked an applicant's class rank (for all 4 years) as number 3 in importance behind rotating at the director's institution and the applicant's USMLE Step 1 score.[1]

FINDING A MENTOR IN YOUR DEPARTMENT OF ORTHOPEDIC SURGERY

Formal exposure to orthopedic surgery during your pre-clinical curriculum years is typically limited. Certainly, the upper and lower extremity portions of gross anatomy give you a taste of the regional anatomy an orthopedic surgeon is invested in on a daily basis. However, a 2002 survey showed that only about 55% of American medical schools required mandatory instruction in musculoskeletal medicine/orthopedic surgery.[2] Therefore, if you are or think you may be interested in orthopedics, you should take the initiative to actively explore and become involved in the field.

Most medical schools offer first-year medical students faculty mentors in various medical or surgical disciplines whom they meet with in order to offer the student the opportunity to shadow these clinicians during clinical encounters. If you are considering orthopedics as a career, then you should consider requesting a clinical mentor in orthopedics to afford yourself early exposure and the opportunity to build your first relationship with your medical school's department of orthopedic surgery. If this opportunity does not exist at your medical school, directly contact a faculty member in the department to request permission to shadow him or her when there is free time in your academic schedule. It is unlikely that an attending will say no to your request. Another option is contacting the residency program director to initiate the process, or discussing approachable faculty members with more senior students or residents. This has the potential to create additional opportunities for you and give you priceless early insights into the field. We must remind you that if you choose to set up a relationship with a clinical mentor, you should follow through on this initiative. Be open about your time limitations and academic schedule. Do not commit to being at office hours or the operating room if you are not absolutely certain you will be there. Attendings and residents have good memories.

GETTING INVOLVED WITH A RESEARCH PROJECT EARLY

An ideal time to gain substantial exposure to the field is during the summer between the first and second years of medical school. At the New York University Hospital for Joint Diseases, we have had tremendous success with our Medical Student Summer Externship for medical students between the first 2 pre-clinical years. This is a highly organized 8-week experience during which the student spends significant time with an assigned faculty mentor and his or her residents of service in the clinic and operating room. Additionally, the students are required to initiate a research project and present their initial progress at the conclusion of the program. Lasting professional relationships are started during this experience from which the committed student can derive further guidance and direction throughout the remaining years of medical school. Forming relationships with the orthopedic residents in the clinical and research settings is invaluable. They, in conjunction with the attending faculty, can give you insights into the field and its subspecialties, afford you additional clinical and research opportunities, and answer questions during the residency application process and about the different types of training programs.

Involvement in a research project is an excellent way to begin to educate oneself about the field, as well as make oneself a more competitive candidate for a residency program. In a 2008 national survey of orthopedic residency program directors, 68% reported that research involvement was a factor in their selection of candidates for interviews.[3] Research started during these summer months should be continued during the second year of medical school. It takes a motivated student who is able to multitask and assume great responsibility to be able to balance the priority of academic excellence in the classroom with the desire to continue to stay meaningfully involved in the orthopedic research he or she has started. Success in these endeavors is certainly recognized by residency selection committees.

Although completing a research project through to publication is a great accomplishment and strengthens your application, please do not think that publication is the only goal when involved in a research project. The learning opportunity itself is invaluable. Additionally, it provides a rare opportunity for you to show the attending your dedication, intelligence, and work ethic. Be ready to do whatever is asked of you and always be a team player. Use this time to network and meet new people. You will be working with residents and attendings who may be in a position to help you one day in a way you cannot see right now. Whether in the form of writing a letter of recommendation or making a phone call, having someone speak positively and genuinely on your behalf can help greatly during the residency application process.

Additionally, the research you conduct does not have to be in the field of orthopedics. Often, applicants have started with interests in other fields, only to be drawn to orthopedics later on in medical school. Commitment to these former research endeavors is valued tremendously and speaks of the character traits of the student applying. Applying for research grants can also help boost your credentials when seeking an orthopedic residency. There are a few ways in which to go about doing this. The National Institutes of Health (NIH) offers research grants to medical students to assist in the funding of a research project (www.training.nih.gov/student). This Summer Research Fellowship is intended to expose students to research that will be conducted either in NIH centers or at your university. Other programs offered by NIH include the Clinical Research Training Program and the Clinical Electives Program for Medical and Dental Students. Information about these programs and other grants can be obtained from the above-referenced Web site or through your medical school. The American Academy of Orthopaedic Surgeons (AAOS) and the Arthroscopy Association of North America (AANA) also supply grant money for medical students. While they are intended primarily for orthopedic residents, you can still apply for these grants with resident and attending sponsorship. (See "Important Contacts" at the end of this chapter, as well as Chapter 12 for more details.) If your time to participate in laboratory research is limited, review papers and retrospective reviews of clinical cohorts are ideal as they allow for the completion of a research project during those times when you are free from medical school obligations (eg, weekends, summers, holidays, and vacations).

USMLE STEP 1

At the end of 2 long years filled with numerous exams, just when you think it is finally over, you are required to take what some call the most important exam of your career thus far. The USMLE Step 1 covers all of the subjects you have studied over the previous 2 years: anatomy, embryology, physiology, immunology, biochemistry, microbiology, pharmacology, pathology, genetics, and the behavioral sciences. It is an 8-hour computer-based exam broken down into 7 sections of 48 questions each. You have 1 hour to complete each section, and a total of 1 hour for breaks between sections, which you can divide up however you choose.

Preparation is critical. It is important to allocate sufficient time for adequate preparation so you do not get overwhelmed. Although there are good review courses that you can take in the few weeks prior to the exam, your USMLE Step 1 preparation should start during your first year. Several review books are available to help you prepare. Among them, and possibly the most well known, is a book titled *First Aid for the USMLE Step 1*. It is an excellent reference and offers high-yield facts that appear on the exam year after year. Champe and Harvey's *Lippincott's Illustrated Reviews: Biochemistry*, Chung and Chung's *Gross Anatomy*, Levinson and Jawetz's *Medical Microbiology & Immunology*, and Fadem's *High-Yield Behavioral Sciences* may also be of use. (See "Recommended Reading" at the end of this chapter.)

Because USMLE Step 1 is computerized, it is essential that you become familiar with and comfortable with taking examinations on the computer. Helpful in this regard is the 15-minute practice test on CD-ROM that you receive when you register for the exam. In addition, several CD-ROM programs are available that feature complete practice board exams, including *Alert: USMLE Step 1*. Many will agree that doing practice questions is one of the best things to do to improve your score. By doing USMLE-style questions early on, you will train your mind to think in a certain way consistently. Usmleworld.com is a very popular resource that students have been using in recent years. This Web site offers you access to more than 2000 USMLE Step 1-style questions that are presented in an interface similar to what you will see on the actual exam. Kaplan's "Q-bank" also offers an online computer-based collection of USMLE-format questions. Other resources are USMLERx.com, the on-site practice test, and the NBME practice test. The more practice questions you do, and the more you understand why you are answering the questions correctly (or more importantly, incorrectly), the better prepared you will be to answer any type of question presented to you on Step 1.

According to a 2008 survey, 75% of orthopedic surgery residency program directors used USMLE Step 1 scores as a factor in their selection of applicants to interview.[2] This is because several studies have correlated performance on USMLE with performance on the Orthopaedics In-Training Exam (OITE). Eighty percent of programs reported that they use a target score as opposed to a passing score only; further, on a scale from 1 to 5, with 1 being not at all important and 5 being very important, the mean rank of the importance of a Step 1 score to program directors was a 4.[2] Accordingly, we cannot stress enough that achieving the highest possible score is crucial for anyone interested in applying to a residency program as competitive as orthopedic surgery. With so many residency selection variables not comparable between medical students, the USMLE is a single metric that allows for the stratification of applicants.

Every year, the National Residency Match Program (NRMP) publishes detailed data on matching statistics including applicants' USMLE Step scores. These data can be found at www.nrmp.org/data/chartingoutcomes2009v3.pdf.

REVIEW COURSES

Depending on the depth of your knowledge and your learning style, you may want to take a classroom- or CD-ROM–based review course for USMLE Step 1. Review courses can range from a commitment of a few days a week to meeting daily for 6 weeks straight. In addition to review courses offered at some medical schools, consider Princeton Review Courses (888-500-PREP, www.princetonreview.com) and Kaplan (800-KAP-TEST, www.kaplanmedical.com), both of which have educational centers nationwide and provide several options in addition to lecture-type courses, including courses and tests on CD-ROM and online courses and/or practice tests on the World Wide Web.

CONCLUSION

Although the first 2 years of medical school can be an overwhelming experience, you should use whatever free time you have to develop relationships in the orthopedic community and become involved in research. This can be particularly beneficial if your research efforts result in publication by the time you apply for an orthopedic residency position. In addition, a letter of recommendation from someone in the orthopedic community who has known you since your first year of medical school will certainly boost your candidacy. Finally, never forget that the most important goal of your first 2 years is to achieve academic excellence, as this is the strongest basis for a successful residency application.

IMPORTANT CONTACTS

Arthroscopy Association of North America (AANA)
6300 North River Road, Suite 104
Rosemont, IL 60018
(847) 292-2262; fax: (847) 292-2268
www.aana.org

American Academy of Orthopaedic Surgeons (AAOS)
6300 North River Road
Rosemont, IL 60018
(847) 823-7186, (800) 346-2267; fax: (847) 823-8031
www.aaos.org

National Institutes of Health (NIH)
Bethesda, MD 20892
www.training.nih.gov/student

Princeton Review Courses
(888) 500-PREP
www.princetonreview.com

Kaplan
(800) KAP-TEST
www.kaplanmedical.com

Usmleworld
www.usmleworld.com

REFERENCES

1. Bernstein AD, Jazrawi LM, Elbeshbeshy B, DellaValle CJ, Zuckerman JD. Orthopedic resident-selection criteria. *J Bone Joint Surg Am.* 2002;84A:2090-2096.
2. Bernstein J, DiCaprio MR, Mehta S. The relationship between required medical school instruction in musculoskeletal medicine and application rates to orthopedic surgery residency programs. *J Bone Joint Surg Am.* 2004;86A:2335-2338.
3. National Resident Matching Program. *Results of the 2008 NRMP Program Director Survey.* 2008. Available at: http://www.nrmp.org/data/programresultsbyspecialty.pdf. Accessed November 17, 2009.

RECOMMENDED READING

Alert: USMLE Step 1. CD-ROM (Win/Mac). New York, NY: McGraw-Hill; 1998.

Champe PC, Harvey RA. *Lippincott's Illustrated Reviews: Biochemistry.* 4th ed. Philadelphia, PA: Lippincott Williams & Wilkins; 2007.

Chung KW, Chung HM. *BRS Gross Anatomy.* 6th ed. Philadelphia, PA: Lippincott Williams & Wilkins; 2007.

Fadem B. *High-Yield Behavioral Sciences.* 3rd ed. Philadelphia, PA: Lippincott Williams & Wilkins; 2008.

Fix JD. *High-Yield Neuroanatomy,* 4th ed. Philadelphia, PA: Lippincott Williams & Wilkins; 2008.

Goljan EF. *Rapid Review Pathology.* 3rd ed. Philadelphia, PA: Mosby; 2009.

Levinson W, Jawetz E. *Medical Microbiology & Immunology: Examination & Board Review.* 8th ed. New York, NY: McGraw-Hill; 2004.

National Resident Matching Program. *Charting Outcomes in the Match: Characteristics of Applicants Who Matched to Their Preferred Specialty in the 2009 NRMP Main Residency Match.* 3rd ed. 2009. Available at: http://www.nrmp.org/data/chartingoutcomes2009v3.pdf. Accessed November 17, 2009.

Sadler TW. *Langmans Medical Embryology.* 11th ed. Philadelphia, PA: Lippincott Williams & Wilkins; 2009.

Tao L, Bhushan V. *First Aid for the USMLE Step 1.* 19th ed. New York, NY: McGraw-Hill Medical; 2008.

Weiss ST. *High-Yield Pharmacology.* Philadelphia, PA: Lippincott Williams & Wilkins; 2009.

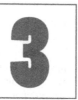

MEDICAL SCHOOL: CLINICAL CLERKSHIPS AND ELECTIVES

After spending 2 long years mostly in the classroom and after taking count-less exams, you finally get an opportunity to apply what you have learned clinically. Although many medical schools are beginning clinical experiences earlier in the cur-riculum, the second 2 years of medical school will be a very novel experience for most. This is the time when you finally begin to feel like a physician, which can be a wonderful experience and give you a taste of what all of the hard work you have put in has been for. However, it is also the time when you need to buckle down and be ready to work harder than ever before.

During the third year, most schools have students rotate through 5 "core" rota-tions. These core rotations include internal medicine, surgery, psychiatry, pediatrics, and obstetrics and gynecology. Different schools dedicate different amounts of time to each, but it is likely that you will spend no less than 6 weeks in each core rotation, with medicine and surgery typically having the longest duration of 8 to 12 weeks.

Knowing that orthopedic surgery is the career path that you would like to pursue, it is important that you do not make the mistake of believing that you can do well on your surgical rotation and then allow your performance to diminish on the other rotations. This should be avoided for a few reasons. First, this will be your primary chance to learn the essentials of medicine as a whole. In almost every clinical scenario that you will be faced with as an orthopedic resident and as an attending surgeon, you will have to consider factors other than the patient's musculoskeletal problem. In addition, as a surgeon, you are ultimately responsible (both ethically and medico-legally) for the health of your patients, and you must be able to assist, if not guide, the medical management of your patients. Although you will probably ask for assistance from colleagues in other specialties in the medical management of your patients, you may be the first line in recognizing and treat-ing your patients' medical problems in the perioperative period and potentially providing life-saving care. In addition, the specialty of orthopedic surgery is practiced everywhere from the newborn nursery to the medical intensive care unit, and your familiarity with managing this wide array of patients will surely impact your overall success as a health care provider. You may only have a few months to learn the basics of these disciplines, so make the most of it! The required clerkships are also important because the selection

---

Lava Y. Patel, BA and Eric J. Strauss, MD

L. M. Jazrawi, K. A. Egol, & J. D. Zuckerman.
Orthopedic Residency & Fellowship: A Guide to Success (pp. 15-22)
© 2010 Taylor & Francis Group

committees of orthopedic surgery residency programs will carefully scrutinize your grades in all of your rotations. Program directors value well-rounded students who demonstrate hard work and consistency during their clerkships. According to a 2008 survey of program directors, grades in required clerkships received a mean importance rating of 4 on a scale of 5 in director's consideration of applicants to interview.[1] In the same survey, consistency of an applicant's grades received a mean importance score of 3.7. Thus, hard work and consistency during your clinical years are critical components of success and are crucial to your development as a physician and as an orthopedic surgeon.

KEYS TO SUCCESS ON THE WARDS

The keys to success on the wards are preparation, hard work, attention to detail, and perseverance. From the moment you arrive at the hospital until the moment you are allowed to leave, you should take every opportunity to learn. You will have a variety of responsibilities during your orthopedic elective/rotation, and managing your time efficiently is very important. You will probably be assigned to a resident and will be expected to do just as he or she does. Morning rounds will usually start anywhere from 5:30 to 6:30 every morning. On certain days, you will be in the operating room all day, and on others, you will spend the majority of the day in clinic. In general, medical students are evaluated based on the "Three As": availability, affability, and ability (in that order of importance).

Availability is the cornerstone of being a good medical student. If you are assigned to work with a specific resident, you should always be with that resident. Although there will be times when your presence is unwanted or you sense you are getting in the way, if your resident is in the hospital, you should be in the hospital. If your resident gets in at 5:00 am for patient rounds, you should be there at 4:45 am. If you are asked to scrub on a case during a surgical rotation, be there early and stay until all of the day's cases are done. When you are done with your cases, ask if there is anything else that you can do to help out. If you want to do well, you should never ask to go home at the end of the day; let your resident or attending tell you to go home. If you know you are going to be spending time in the OR the next day, make sure you know what procedures you will be scrubbing into so that you can go home and read about them in more detail. As a medical student, knowledge of the relevant anatomy and surgical approach are often the keys to understanding what is going on in the OR and will allow you to be prepared in the event that the attending "pimps" you during the case.

There is nothing worse to an attending or resident than medical students who are nowhere to be found when they are wanted or needed. Even if the rotation you are on is not your main interest, hard work will always pay off in terms of gaining knowledge and experience. Those with whom you will work find it more rewarding to be working with and teaching a medical student who is inquisitive, eager to learn, and excited about being in the hospital taking care of patients. Every task in which you participate, from drawing blood to removing sutures, has some value with regard to learning efficient and effective patient care. Also, remember that you may have a limited window of time to learn the basics and art of medicine. Don't cheat yourself out of this experience.

Regarding the second "A," affability, grading on these types of rotations can be very subjective. If you are well liked by those around you and work well as a member of the team, you have a better chance of receiving a good evaluation. Although it is difficult to give firm recommendations on how to be "affable," some basic guidelines are worth mentioning. The first is that no one likes to be around a complainer. You should be helpful and happy about being in the hospital taking care of patients. This is truly a unique privilege that should be respected. No matter what the task, make sure you are always available and willing to do whatever is asked of you. At the same time, do not be afraid to ask questions, as residents/attendings will be some of your best resources.

If at any point you get the urge to complain or feel grumpy—even if you have been up all night—just think, "I could be studying for a pharmacology exam!" The most difficult part of being liked on a rotation is balancing your desire to be "available" against the tendency to appear pushy. Try to get a feel for those you work with and for what works and what doesn't work. Be helpful and friendly, but don't overdo it. Be polite and respectful. If the residents are acting informally with an attending or colleague, try not to get caught up in their familiarity, as this can make you appear too comfortable. Orthopedic surgery is a highly competitive specialty with directors looking for reasons to deny an interview; don't give them a reason to reject your application. Remember that you are part of a team. While competition between medical students exists during a rotation, attendings and residents pick up on students who act only in their own best interests. Teamwork is a mantra we live by; those who do not respect this tenet at this level will find it even harder to do so further along their training. A final suggestion is to remember that you are on the lowest rung of the ladder, and so sometimes it is better to speak only when spoken to.

On the third "A," ability, there is a certain amount of basic knowledge that must be acquired during your required clerkships; as previously stated, it is important to master this body of information both for your evaluations and for your future as a physician. The key to acquiring the necessary knowledge for any given rotation is having the right resources. Speak to students who have rotated before you and to the residents on your team to find out which textbooks, journal articles, and Web sites work best for building a foundation of knowledge. Once you have the right resources, the basic tenet that hard work leads to success prevails once again. If you are assigned a patient with tuberculosis to follow on your medicine rotation, make sure you read on that topic the night before you are going to present the patient to the senior resident or attending during rounds. While this advice might seem obvious, one is continually surprised when a student who is assigned to scrub on a laparoscopic cholecystectomy does not prepare with at least the basic background of the topic and the relevant anatomy. Your clinical rotations are like one big open-book test; prepare for rounds and conferences, and you will do well. If you are on a surgical rotation, do not leave the hospital until you know what cases are scheduled in the room that you are assigned to so that you can adequately prepare yourself on the appropriate topics.

Another key to performing well is to carry a good handbook with you. If you see a patient in clinic or are asked to scrub on a case that you did not know about the night before, read a little so that you have some familiarity with the subject matter. Even a quick Internet search 10 minutes before a case will provide you with some useful information. One of the benefits to diligent work during these rotations is that the second part of the United States Medical Licensing Examination (USMLE) will be a breeze if you have mastered the basics during your required clinical rotations. A topic that falls under ability and may lead to undue stress is manual dexterity. Your resident will not care if you couldn't place that intravenous line or draw an arterial blood gas. If you can, it is a bonus. If you are asked to do something and cannot complete the task, be honest and let the person in charge know. Try to do as many procedures as you can while a student because before you know it, you will be expected to perform many of these procedures as an intern. The more comfortable you are with simple procedures at that time, the better off you will be later. Last, do not appear disinterested at any time during your rotation. Most importantly, as stated previously, be dependable; never disappear.

ALPHA OMEGA ALPHA

In addition, your performance in these rotations may also weigh heavily into determining your acceptance into Alpha Omega Alpha (AΩA), the medical students' honor society, which is another important criterion that residency directors use to select orthopedic surgery residents. In the 2008 National Resident Matching Program (NRMP) Program Directors Survey, 75% of program directors reported looking for AΩA membership in potential applicants.[1,2]

ELECTIVE ROTATIONS

During the end of the third year and into the fourth year, you will be permitted to choose elective rotations. For those of you who are interested in a surgical subspecialty, such as orthopedic surgery, these electives can be a great opportunity for you to excel and to show that you are a competitive potential applicant.

Your elective rotations should:

- ✓ Help you make a career decision
- ✓ Round out your education
- ✓ Provide you with a close working relationship with senior residents and attendings who can write you letters of recommendation
- ✓ Give you a feel for how different residency programs are organized and run (large academic centers compared to smaller community programs)

Although the specifics on letters of recommendation are covered in Chapter 6, some basics will be covered here as well. As far as being successful in these rotations, the previously outlined recommendations apply. If you are completing a specific rotation primarily to obtain a letter, working hard is going to be the key to success. The first thing your elective rotations should accomplish is helping you decide which type of residency you want to pursue. For some of us, this decision is relatively easy; for others, this is much more difficult. Make sure to schedule the elective rotations that are going to help you make these decisions early as some residency programs participate in an "early match," and you don't want to be left out in the cold should you change your mind. These electives, as previously stated, should also serve to "round out" your educational background. Every applicant to orthopedic programs should complete a subinternship in general surgery. This rotation will help hone your knowledge on perioperative patient management. In addition, students often get their first opportunity here to first-assist on cases and learn the basics of wound closure.

Subinternships in internal medicine, emergency medicine, radiology, and anesthesia are often useful and should be strongly considered by applicants to orthopedic surgery programs. Your final goal for elective rotations is obtaining letters of recommendation—optimally, standout letters. A letter that describes you as "the best medical student in 5 years" will go a long way toward making you stand out from your peers (and other applicants). These letters are particularly helpful when they are read by an individual who knows the writer. When selecting among orthopedic rotations, try to find out which attendings are medical student advocates, and then do everything in your power to work with these individuals. Keep in mind that the "big name" attendings may not be the biggest student advocates and may not help you obtain a residency position no matter how good a medical student you are. The only way to find out which attendings are student advocates is by talking to students in the year(s) ahead of you and to residents within the department; their insights can be invaluable. In addition, if the biggest student advocate is a foot and ankle surgeon, do that rotation whether or not you have any interest in foot and ankle surgery. Once you have decided on orthopedic surgery, the content of any given rotation is almost irrelevant. The key is to work hard and to get to know the attending so he or she can support your efforts for residency training.

HOME ROTATION

In 2008, 84% of orthopedic residency program directors reported that they use audition electives as a factor in selecting applicants to interview.[3] You should make an informed decision whether to choose an elective in orthopedics and, if so, whether to choose a home or away rotation. The differences in home and away rotations are discussed next.

Choosing an orthopedic surgery elective at your home hospital is a good place to start for numerous reasons. First, certain schools may favor their own students during interview season. Second, doing an elective at your own school will give you access to different attendings who may be involved in the residency selection process. This can be an invaluable opportunity for you to show them your dedication, knowledge base, and work ethic. You should also do your best to build a close working relationship with at least one attending who will be able to write you a strong letter of recommendation when the time comes. We also advise that you introduce yourself to the chairman of the department at the very beginning of your rotation or at your earliest opportunity. Take some time to let him or her know that you are interested in orthopedics and plan to apply for a residency position in the upcoming match season.

AWAY ROTATIONS

How to Choose

Many students interested in orthopedic surgery elect to do rotations at other institutions. These away rotations allow you to learn more about a specific program you may be interested in. There is no better way to learn about a program than spending time working with residents. They will tell you exactly how good their experiences are and how happy they are with their training.

Another reason for completing an away rotation is to enhance your chances of matching at that program. Certain programs preferably or even exclusively interview candidates who have rotated on one of their services. If you are interested in a particular program, it is worth investigating that program's track record in terms of interviewing students who have completed rotations with them. This information may be difficult to find and may entail calling previous graduates from your medical school who have rotated there. It is important to keep in mind, however, that while an away rotation can help your chances of matching at a particular program, it can also hurt you. In a new and unfamiliar environment, you may not be able to perform quite as well. In addition, if you have a problem with a particular attending, resident, or support staff member while on such a rotation, your chances of matching may be severely hampered because they have only a limited experience with you.

It is important for third- and fourth-year students to be familiar with the types of orthopedic programs available at other schools/hospitals. Most, if not all, programs are considered either community programs or academic programs. The academic programs are affiliated with certain medical schools and tend to have a number of affiliated hospitals at which you would potentially rotate. These programs tend to be larger and offer more first-year positions than the community-based programs. The community-based programs tend to be smaller in size, to be affiliated with fewer hospitals, and to have a fewer number of available positions.

How to Succeed

Consider scheduling the rotation that is most desirable for you last. The previous orthopedic electives will provide you with a knowledge base that will allow you to shine during this rotation. If you decide to do an away rotation, the rules for success are the same as those previously given: work harder than everyone around you, be well prepared for your cases and conferences, and always be extra polite, because everyone can help or hurt you—including nurses, scrub techs, and office staff.

RESEARCH ELECTIVES

Many schools offer their students the opportunity to participate in a research elective. Time commitments may vary, but they usually involve students spending a couple of weeks doing research at an institution rather than clinical training. If you are in your fourth year of medical school, participating in a research project has many potential benefits. During your research elective, you will be provided with the time and resources necessary to complete a clinical or basic science study. This experience will be valuable with regard to increasing your knowledge about the topic that you are investigating, in addition to gaining the skills and experience vital to being successful in this era where evidence-based medicine is becoming increasingly important. As many academic residency programs have research requirements for their residents, having this experience as a medical student will give you a leg up on your peers who have not had this opportunity. If possible, do your best to get involved in writing up the research activity that you participate in. Publications on a medical student's residency application are regarded highly and provide a good topic for discussion during your interview. Last, a research experience allows for the opportunity to make an impression on the principal investigator and other members of the department, showing that your level of dedication and work ethic extends beyond your efforts in the clinical setting.

EXTRACURRICULAR ACTIVITIES

Participation in clubs and interest groups as a medical student helps round out your education and shows that you are more than just grades and test scores. These experiences can be valuable in many ways and are definitely encouraged. Keep in mind that your involvement should be about quality and not quantity. Rather than joining numerous clubs and becoming a member, join one or two that you are passionate about and be intimately involved in those. Program directors would much rather see applicants who have leadership roles in organizations and involvement in charitable endeavors rather than those who are just "members" of many organizations and clubs.

REFERENCES

1. National Resident Matching Program. *Results of the 2008 NRMP Program Director Survey.* 2008. Available at: http://www.nrmp.org/data/programresultsbyspecialty.pdf. Accessed November 17, 2009.

2. National Resident Matching Program. *Charting Outcomes in the Match: Characteristics of Applicants Who Matched to Their Preferred Specialty in the 2009 NRMP Main Residency Match.* 3rd ed. 2009. Available at: http://www.nrmp.org/data/chartingoutcomes2009v3.pdf. Accessed November 17, 2009.

3. Yeh AC, Franko O, Day CS. Impact of clinical electives and residency interest on medical students' education in musculoskeletal medicine. *J Bone Joint Surg Am.* 2008;90(2): 307-315.

THE APPLICATION PROCESS

Making the decision to pursue a career in orthopedic surgery is the easy part. Now comes the tough part. You must concentrate all of your efforts on making your application look attractive to residency programs. The application process is the key step in achieving your goal of becoming an orthopedic surgeon and is the culmination of all of your hard work up to this point. Unless you have done an away rotation at an institution or it is your home institution, your application is the first impression that program directors have of you. Along with your board scores and recommendations, your application will help programs decide whether to consider you as a candidate and take the next step of inviting you for an interview. A strong application is what gets your "foot in the door," and therefore it is so important that it be optimized. The application process can be daunting, but adhering to a few basic principles can facilitate the process and increase your chances of getting into the program of your choice. This chapter will go through these principles as well as how to put it all together in the actual application.

As with all things in life, *timing* is everything. Orthopedics is an extremely competitive field, so once you have considered it as a possible career path, it is important to start shaping your application and gathering information about programs and the application process. You should find an advisor to give you some guidance. There may be an "orthopedic surgery club" at your medical school that can help guide you to the proper people. Senior medical students who have recently gone through the process can give you the latest information on the application process, interviews, and programs. Orthopedic residents and faculty at your home institution or during your away electives can also offer excellent insight into what programs are looking for and what it takes to get into residency. The chairperson of your institution is another invaluable resource as he or she can give you a firsthand account of what he or she feels is the most important part of the application and his or her opinion on other programs. Often, your dean's office will assign you an advisor. However, if one is not assigned, it is important to find an advisor in the orthopedics department so you can learn more about the field and start shaping your application. Table 4-1 provides a timeline that can help you plan for the application process.

Crispin C. Ong, MD and David E. Ruchelsman, MD

L. M. Jazrawi, K. A. Egol, & J. D. Zuckerman.
Orthopedic Residency & Fellowship: A Guide to Success (pp. 23-32)
© 2010 Taylor & Francis Group.

Table 4-1

APPLICATION TIMELINE FOR
ORTHOPEDIC RESIDENCY PROGRAMS

THIRD YEAR

January	• Find an advisor in your orthopedic surgery department.
February	• Begin thinking about fourth-year electives. Decide when you will rotate at your home institution and select away rotations.
March/April	• Gather information about the different programs and familiarize yourself with the application process. Use all of your resources: chairperson, residents, advisor, senior medical students, program Web sites, etc.
May	• Request application materials and information from a large number and variety of programs. • Make note of deadlines and any special requirements.
June	• Start writing a draft of your personal statement.
July	• MyERAS Web site opens to applicants. Contact your dean's office for ERAS processing instructions and to receive your Electronic Residency Application Service (ERAS) token. • Familiarize yourself with the content of ERAS by downloading the MyERAS application worksheet and user guide. Begin working on your application. • This is also a good time to ask selected faculty members whom you have worked with closely and who know you well for letters of recommendation (remember to ask early). • Keep working on that personal statement. Have your advisor or someone else you trust review your personal statement and give you suggestions and criticism.
August	• Register with the National Residency Matching Program (NRMP) (www.nrmp.org) so that you can participate in the Match. (Note: This is a separate process from ERAS.) • Have an application photograph taken if you don't already have one. • Confirm that letters of recommendation have been sent. • Put the finishing touches on your personal statement. • If applying to non-ERAS institutions, request that transcripts, letters of recommendation, and United States Medical Licensing Examination (USMLE) scores be sent.

FOURTH YEAR

September/ October	• Complete, certify, and submit your ERAS application on the Internet, and submit your non-ERAS applications as well. • Check the status of your application by using the Applicant Document Tracking System (ADTS) and monitor the message center for information from the programs to which you applied. Continue to check ADTS to confirm that your application is complete. You have to follow-up on items such as letters of recommendation and your dean's letter that are not under your control. • Verify that your non-ERAS applications are complete. • Keep your profile up to date, as programs will contact you based on the information (email, address, phone) on your ERAS application.
October/ November	• Programs begin to extend invitations to interview. Schedule your interviews as soon as you are invited, as spots are assigned on a first-come, first-served basis. • Dean's letter is typically sent in the beginning of November.

Table 4-1 (continued)

APPLICATION TIMELINE FOR
ORTHOPEDIC RESIDENCY PROGRAMS

FOURTH YEAR

November–January	• Attend interviews and send thank you letters. • Think about your rank list. Assess each institution you visit and ask yourself if you would be happy there.
February	• Submit your rank list on the NRMP Web site. • Sit back, relax, and wait for the results.
March	• Unmatch day: Usually the Monday preceding match day, when those who have not matched find out via an NRMP email and/or dean's office. • Scramble day: Usually the Tuesday preceding match day, when those who have not matched "scramble" for a residency position. • Match day: Usually a Thursday, when match results are distributed by your dean's office and the NRMP Web site.

Being on time, or preferably early, is important at every step in the process. It is never too early to start gathering information about different programs, as residencies may have different requirements and deadlines. Letters of recommendation should be requested far in advance of application deadlines as your letter writers may ask you to provide them with additional information and may also be pressed to write letters for other students. Asking your letter writers early not only gives them ample time to write you a thoughtful letter, but is also a matter of courtesy. Also, it may be obvious, but submitting your application on time or preferably early and being punctual to interviews is extremely important. So, whether it's gathering information about the field of orthopedics and different residency programs, finding an advisor in the application process, or completing your actual application, starting early is the key to a successful application.

Organization is another integral part of the application process. There is a lot of information available about different programs, and it is important to keep track of it. The American Medical Association (AMA) maintains the Fellowship and Residency Electronic Interactive Database (FREIDA, https://freida.ama-assn.org/Freida/user/viewProgramSearch.do), which lists all of the orthopedic residency programs approved by the Accreditation Council of Graduate Medical Education (ACGME). This is a good starting place to learn about the basics of programs such as contact information, application requirements, program size, work schedule, educational environment, and employment policies and benefits. The site also has links to individual residency programs that often have more detailed information about the program and application requirements. The ERAS site (www.aamc.org/students/eras) also has useful contact information. You should also request information from the individual residency programs you are interested in the summer before you apply, as it is important to keep abreast of the most current requirements and deadlines.

Keeping yourself organized is even more critical when you start to accumulate the different parts of your application and get ready to submit it. You should keep a record of what information you send individual programs and when your interview is scheduled.

Keeping organized will help you to get your application in on time (or better yet, early), to decide what programs interest you, to prepare for interviews as you approach the interview season, and to help you make your rank list.

Once you master the first 2 principles of timing and organization, then it's time for some *introspection*. To successfully get into an orthopedic residency, you have to ask yourself what kind of residency program you would be happy with and which programs match your credentials and attributes. You must ask yourself the following important questions and answer them as honestly as possible:

✓ *How competitive an applicant am I?* Program directors look at a number of factors when evaluating a candidate at the initial stages of the application process. They take into account things such as grades, board scores, research experience, letters of recommendation, honors/awards, and Alpha Omega Alpha (AΩA) membership to name a few. If there are aspects of your application that are deficient, it is important to take this into consideration when deciding the number of programs to apply to and which programs to apply to. Your advisor or the program director of your home institution can give you an objective view on how competitive a candidate you are.

✓ *What factors are most important to me in choosing a residency program?* A variety of factors influence your decision to choose a particular program. Here are a few important things to consider (this topic is addressed in more detail in the section on Choosing a Residency Program):

   o *Size:* Programs vary in size anywhere from 2 to 14 residents per class. Do I want to be part of a larger program, which may have more resources, a larger faculty, and a wider variety of colleagues with whom to work? Or, on the opposite extreme, do I want a smaller program with a handful of residents who I will get to know and work closely with for the next 5 years?

   o *Academic environment:* What kind of learning environment would suit me best? Do I want a program that stresses academics with frequent didactics and conferences or one that is less structured?

   o *Research:* Am I interested in pursuing clinical/basic science research? Do I want a program that emphasizes research as part of its curriculum? Are there opportunities and resources available for residents to perform research?

   o *Location:* Do I have any geographic preference for where I do my residency (city versus small town versus rural areas)? Do I have any geographical constraints? Getting into an orthopedic residency is extremely competitive, so it is best not to limit yourself too much in this respect. However, it is also important to consider where you would be happy living as you will have to spend the next 5 years of your life there.

Asking yourself these questions and answering honestly will make deciding which particular programs to apply to more manageable. You must match what you want from a program with realistic expectations of your chances of getting into a particular program with your credentials. You should apply to 25 to 45 programs depending on your level of competitiveness, and you should apply to a variety of programs. Your only limitation is the cost of applications because applying to different programs on ERAS is as simple as an additional mouse-click. While applying to more programs may cost more, in the long run, this is a small price to pay for increasing your chances of obtaining a residency position.

Furthermore, because getting an orthopedic residency position is extremely competitive, it is important to be strategic when applying. You should use the information you have gathered thus far on programs to determine which programs are most competitive, moderately competitive, and least competitive, and apply to several programs in each class to diversify your chances. And, no matter how competitive an applicant you think you may be, do not make the mistake of applying to only the most competitive programs (unless you are prepared not to match). You can always decline an interview, but you can't be extended an interview if you haven't applied. Introspection is important throughout the application process and is also important when you have to decide on your rank list. When that time comes, you will have to review all of the information you have gathered from interviews, advisors, tours on the interview trail, and the gut feeling you got when you met with the faculty and residents of the various programs to figure out where you will be the happiest when doing your training.

Finally, perhaps the most important principle of a successful application is *professionalism*. This principle should permeate all aspects of the application process. Everything you do, from requesting information from programs to writing thank you letters, should be refined as it is a reflection of your character. Courtesy and respect should be extended to everyone you have contact with from the program secretary to chairperson. Now, it should go without saying, but professionalism also includes representing yourself accurately in your application. Be prepared to answer questions on anything that you include in your application. Put forth the best representation of yourself on paper, but always be honest.

THE APPLICATION–ERAS

Now that you have the basic principles down, it's time to discuss the details of the application itself. Almost all orthopedic residency programs use ERAS, sponsored by the American Association of Medical Colleges (AAMC, www.aamc.org/students/eras). ERAS is an online service that transmits applications, letters of recommendation, Medical Student Performance Evaluations (MSPEs), medical school transcripts, USMLE transcripts, Comprehensive Osteopathic Medical Licensing Examination (COMLEX) transcripts, and other supporting credentials from you and your designated dean's office to program directors using the Internet. ERAS consists of MyERAS (the Web site where you create your application), the dean's office workstation, the program director's workstation, and the ERAS PostOffice. It is used by all medical schools in the United States, the Canadian Resident Matching Service, and the Educational Commission for Foreign Medical Graduates (ECFMG). The ERAS application includes the following documents:

- ✓ Common application form (CAF), which is comprised of the information in both the profile and application
- ✓ Personal statement
- ✓ MSPE (aka, dean's letter)
- ✓ Letters of recommendation
- ✓ Medical School Transcript
- ✓ USMLE transcript
- ✓ COMLEX transcript (osteopathic medical graduates only)
- ✓ ECFMG status report (international medical graduates only)
- ✓ Wallet-sized color photograph

Once you have gathered enough information about the different programs you are interested in by using all of the aforementioned resources (with emphasis on deadlines and requirements), you can start your ERAS application. The following steps are referenced from the ERAS Web site:

1. Obtain a token—an alphanumeric code used to register and access MyERAS online—from your dean's office (if you are a foreign medical graduate, contact the ECFMG). Register and access MyERAS using your AAMC ID. The ERAS Web site has a MyERAS user guide and worksheet that is helpful.

2. Complete the CAF and personal statement(s) using MyERAS. You will be asked to provide information about your education, awards/honors, research/work/volunteer experiences, publications, USMLE scores, and extracurricular interests. You will also be asked to input your personal statement (see following sections for more details).

3. Specify the programs to which you wish to apply, and assign documents (eg, letters of recommendation, personal statement) to specific programs. Your application materials will be transmitted from the ERAS PostOffice.

4. Review your application carefully before certification. Review your application for any misspellings, omissions, and discrepancies. You may only certify and submit your application once! And once you have submitted your application, you will not be able to make any changes to it or update any information on your CAF. Certify and submit. Submitting your application prompts your dean's office to transmit your supporting documents (eg, dean's letter, letters of recommendation, photograph, and medical school transcripts) to the ERAS PostOffice and the National Board of Medical Examiners to transmit your USMLE transcript to the ERAS PostOffice.

5. Track the delivery of documents to the programs through the ADTS and monitor the message center for information from residency programs and important notices from ERAS including information on billing and the Scramble. Programs will contact you using the mailing address, email address, and/or telephone number that you provide on your application, so make sure this information is up-to-date and that you check your mail and messages frequently.

The application process may seem confusing, so it is important to start early (*Timing* is everything, and being *organized* helps too!). The ERAS PostOffice opens in early September, so you should aim to submit your materials by that time, even though your letters of recommendation, dean's letter, and medical school transcript will probably not yet be available. Note that you do not have to certify/submit your application in the same session in which you enter information. If you anticipate needing to update any section of your ERAS application, you may "save" your session and either update your personal information or specify additional programs at any time before certification. Help using the ERAS system can be obtained from the "Resources to Download" tab on the ERAS Web site and by consulting with your dean's office, residents, and senior medical students. Make sure that you include all important pieces of information somewhere in your application, curriculum vitae (CV), or personal statement. Often, the application is the first impression program directors are exposed to, so you should put your best foot forward and highlight your achievements.

In addition to ERAS, some programs have additional requirements. They may request that you provide them with a CV, college transcripts, MCAT scores, supplemental application forms, particular requirements for letters of recommendation, and special parameters for your personal statement. Getting this information can take some time and legwork, so it is important to find out early. Some of these requirements may be listed on FREIDA or the residency program's Web site. Keep an organized record of what you have sent each program and follow up to make sure the program received it.

There are a few orthopedic programs that use non-ERAS applications, but these are rare. If you decide to apply to these programs, be sure to request application information early, make sure that all supporting documents (eg, dean's letters, medical school transcripts, letters of recommendation, and USMLE transcripts) are sent to the program along with your application, and confirm that the program received the documents you sent.

THE PHOTOGRAPH

You will need to provide a wallet-sized portrait photo of yourself for your ERAS application. If you do not have an appropriate photograph of yourself in professional attire, now is the time to have one taken. Avoid photos that you feel "make you look good" if they have you unshaven, unkempt, or inappropriately attired. Submit one print to your dean's office, and they will upload it to the ERAS PostOffice along with your other documents. Some programs request additional photographs that they may use to help remember you when interviewing and ranking you, so it's a good idea to order several prints. Furthermore, you may also need a photo when you start your residency to make a face sheet for resident identification. The usual size of photos requested is approximately 2.5 x 3.5 inches and not more than 3 x 4 inches.

THE PERSONAL STATEMENT

The personal statement is the part of the application process that causes the most stress for applicants. The rest of your application simply states the facts. The personal statement is a means to convey the things that are not outlined in the rest of your application. There is no recommended topic, so it is up to you to decide what to write about. Some programs request that you include specific information in your personal statement. If this is the case, then you should address their questions somewhere in your statement.

The personal statement should not simply be a summary of your application but should be used to show your motivation, dedication, and deliberate progress toward your goal of becoming an orthopedic surgeon as well as to highlight anything that makes you interesting or special. Some suggest using the personal statement to explain unflattering aspects of your application, such as poor grades in a particular subject. Others recommend against this, arguing that this will only unnecessarily highlight a negative aspect of your application. Unless there is a compelling reason, I believe that your statement should focus on the positive aspects of your application, but you should always consult your advisor.

Here are some questions that you might want to address in your statement:

- ✓ Why are you pursuing a career in orthopedic surgery? Why are you particularly suited for this field?
- ✓ What special leadership abilities do you have, and what have you done to exemplify them? What have you overcome to get here?

✓ What are your major research accomplishments and interests? Do you plan to pursue research in the future?

✓ What is your passion? What makes you interesting? How much more of you is there beyond the numbers and grades that are found in your application?

✓ Do you pursue extracurricular activities? Do you have a life outside of the classroom and off the wards?

✓ What are you looking for in a residency program? What do you plan to do in the future? Private practice, Academics, or something else?

As you begin to write your personal statement, here are some important things to keep in mind:

✓ *Start early.* The personal statement is the part of your application that is likely to require the most time and effort. If you are not a good writer, you should try to organize your ideas and use a style guide such as *Strunk and White's Elements of Style*, now in its 4th edition; an online version of the original 1918 edition appears at www.bartleby.com/141. (See also Appendix B.) You should also have many people review your personal statement and get their opinion on style and content.

✓ *Limit it to one page.* Program directors have to read hundreds of personal statements, so it is important to be straightforward and to the point. Try to make your statement interesting, but by no means should you try to be too creative, use gimmicks, or write about something that is totally off-the-wall. A conventional (even if boring) personal statement is better than a wacky one that makes you stand out in the wrong way. Program directors have so many candidates and so few residency spots that they are just looking for reasons to eliminate people from their list.

✓ *Revise, proofread, revise, proofread, etc.* The personal statement provides insight to the kind of person you are beyond the credentials and scores in the rest of your application, so it is important that you make a good impression. Create your personal statement(s) using a word processor, perform a spell check, and then cut and paste the text into ERAS (be aware of any formatting changes that may be altered or lost by this action). Use standard spelling and grammar. Proofread and revise your personal statement meticulously, and have others do it as well. Poor grammar, misspellings, and typographical errors are red flags that can easily be avoided.

✓ *Represent yourself honestly.* This goes back to the basic principle of professionalism. Anything you write in your personal statement (and application for that matter) is fair game. Be prepared to talk about anything you mention in your statement. There should not be any discrepancies between what program directors/interviewers read in your statement and how you are in person.

ERAS allows you to create one or more personal statements and assign them to different programs. This can be helpful if you wish to personalize your statement or if a particular program has length restrictions or content guidelines.

THE CURRICULUM VITAE

ERAS currently has a function that formats your application into a CV format; however, some programs may still ask you to submit a CV with your application. If you already have a CV, you should revise and update it. If you don't have one, now is a good time to make one. Your CV should provide a snapshot of your educational, professional, and extracurricular activities and accomplishments along with your basic personal information. Similar to your personal statement, it should be clear, straightforward, readable, and ideally fit on one page (unless you have extensive work experience or a long list of publications).

Use efficient headings, accurate titles, and descriptions. Tailor your CV to your target audience, and explain any activity that is not clear from its name with a short description. Use action verbs, and avoid the passive voice. Use the same principles for writing your personal statement: start early; be concise and accurate; meticulously proofread/revise and have your advisor, dean's office, as well as others proofread/revise; and be honest and professional.

Here are some suggested section headings in no particular order:

- ✓ Personal information: name, address, phone number, email address
- ✓ Education (starting with college): school(s), degree(s), test scores, GPA/class rank, awards/honors
- ✓ Publications/presentations
- ✓ Research experience
- ✓ Work experience
- ✓ Military service
- ✓ Language skills
- ✓ Extracurricular activities and interests
- ✓ Professional memberships

In conclusion, the application process is the means by which you convey to programs your accomplishments and motivation for your pursuit of orthopedics as a career. Adhering to the principles we started with at the beginning of this chapter (timing, organization, introspection, and professionalism) can help facilitate the application process and hopefully can help you achieve a successful match.

LETTERS OF RECOMMENDATION

Much has changed since the last edition of this book. My role has now changed from writing and editing the book as an orthopedic resident to writing and editing as an orthopedic attending. As I write this chapter and reflect on the writing of the first edition, not much has changed in the overall application process other than minor changes in the format and deadlines. Grades, test scores, and affability still remain paramount in the selection process. Advice for this remains the same and is detailed in other chapters. During this process, you have perfected your curriculum vitae (CV) and labored over writing a personal statement that will not appear outlandish. Finally, to complete your application prior to the interview, you will need to ask for letters in support of your application (ie, letters of recommendation).

Orthopedics continues to remain one of the most competitive subspecialties. Most applicants continue to be Alpha Omega Alpha (AΩA) or its equivalent and scored 99% on the boards. Letters of recommendation highlight traits that cannot be seen in the CV, personal statement, or transcript. These traits include, but are not limited to, reliability, work ethic, and the ability to work well with others. The letter of recommendation will be the reviewer's only window into how others subjectively assess your personality and whether you would be a good fit for their program. The most common questions during this process include the following: How many letters do I need? Who should I ask for a letter? When should I ask for a letter? How should I ask for a letter? What should I provide the writer with? The inspiration for this revised chapter continues to be Basil Elbeshbeshy, MD, author of the first edition chapter on recommendation letters. Much of what he wrote about almost 10 years ago remains true today. At the time, he was a fellow orthopedic resident. In addition to that perspective, I will include my views as an orthopedic attending involved in the process of selecting new residents for our program.

HOW MANY LETTERS DO I NEED?

First, you will have your dean's letter. You have little control over this letter. Basically, the dean of your school will review your folder and formulate a summary of

Laith M. Jazrawi, MD

L. M. Jazrawi, K. A. Egol, & J. D. Zuckerman.
Orthopedic Residency & Fellowship: A Guide to Success (pp. 33-36)
© 2010 Taylor & Francis Group.

your medical school performance from the first 2 years and your clinical clerkships. Comments from your preceptors and often senior residents' comments on your performance will be included. So, in other words, try to get along with everyone on your service during your clinical clerkships. The dean will usually meet briefly with you before preparing the letter so that your background can be included in the letter. This letter will also be used to address any unusual circumstances, such as a leave of absence. A dean's letter typically concludes with a summary statement rating your overall qualifications as an applicant for postgraduate training ("outstanding," "excellent," "superior," etc) that provides a means of comparing you to your classmates. A statement regarding your ranking in the class will also be included. This is the most important part of the letter; generally, the rest is cookbook in nature and difficult to use as a basis for distinguishing between applicants.

In addition to your dean's letter, you will almost definitely need a letter from the chairperson of your school's department of orthopedics or the orthopedic residency program director. If it is specifically required, its absence may raise a red flag. It should be requested upon completion of your clinical elective in orthopedics. Even if you did not work directly with either of these individuals, they will summarize the comments of the residents and other attendings with whom you worked.

Beyond these two letters, you are free to ask for recommendations from whomever you wish. Keep in mind that reviewers are usually overwhelmed with paperwork and may be put off by having to read more than four letters. The Electronic Residency Application Service (ERAS) also limits the total number of letters you can submit to four. Applicants should visit www.aamc.org/students/eras/resources/start.htm for detailed instructions regarding letters of recommendation. Bottom line: unless you have a compelling reason, limit your letters of recommendation to four—and, of course, never submit more than the limit specified by any program.

WHOM SHOULD I ASK FOR A LETTER?

In deciding whom to ask for letters (in addition to the dean and chairperson of orthopedics), several factors must be considered. First and foremost, the letter writer should know you personally and should have worked with you in some fashion. As stated previously, these letters ideally serve to inform the reviewer regarding aspects of you not found in your folder; such knowledge can only be obtained from someone who knows you and has worked with you. Savvy reviewers read letters looking for some indication of the circumstances under which the writer got to know you. Name recognition alone should not be a factor in choosing whom to ask for a letter. Don't ask a "big name" in your school's orthopedic department for a letter if you haven't worked with him or her.

Second, you should be certain that the writer has a positive impression of you. If you are not sure, or if you sense that he or she is not entirely comfortable writing you a letter, ask someone else! Nothing will sink you faster than a negative remark in a letter of recommendation—or even an equivocal comment.

You may also ask for a letter from a researcher with whom you have worked extensively. If you have spent time on an away rotation, ask a chief or senior resident to write a letter for your file at that school. While it may not carry significant weight at other institutions, a positive letter from a senior resident at the institution to which you are applying can go a long way in convincing higher-ups that you are a good fit for the program. Letters should come from orthopedic attendings when possible, rather than non-orthopedic attendings. Still, it is better to get a superlative letter from a non-orthopedic attending (with phrases like "outstanding" and "the best student I can remember") than a lukewarm letter from an orthopedist. Finally, some institutions will request a letter from the chief resident. These letters should generally be sent only to institutions that request them.

WHEN SHOULD I ASK FOR A LETTER?

As a courtesy to the writer, when requesting a letter, you should attempt to give as much advance notice as possible. If you are doing a rotation with that person, ask for the letter near the end of the rotation or immediately after completion while your performance is still fresh in his or her mind. Performing a clinical elective in orthopedics at your medical school early in your fourth year maximizes the potential to receive your letters in a timely fashion. This needs to be balanced by using early orthopedic electives as preparation for electives at your desired orthopedic residency training program.

HOW SHOULD I ASK FOR A LETTER?

If you performed well on a rotation and were well liked by a certain attending, then asking for the letter should be quite simple. In general, writers of recommendation letters are eager to support an applicant who they feel will genuinely be a good resident. If you have chosen your letter writers wisely, then asking for the letters is the easy part. Requesting the letter should be done verbally and followed up by a formal letter or email. Once again, if there is any reluctance or hesitation on the writer's part, ask someone else.

WHAT SHOULD I PROVIDE THE WRITER WITH?

Feel free to give the writer whatever documentation you think will be helpful. Your personal statement and CV are usually sufficient, along with a list of the programs that you will be applying to; the ERAS system can generate a list of the latter. The system can also generate a formal letter requesting a letter of recommendation. Stay away from the CVs generated by the ERAS system: they are formatted in a list form that is difficult to read. Provide letter writers with your personalized CV and personal statement and the ERAS letter requesting a letter of recommendation. Your letters of recommendation should be sent to ERAS to be scanned into their system so that program directors at the institutions to which you apply can visit the Web site and view the appropriate documents.

Make the writing/mailing process as painless as possible for your letter writers—more specifically, for their clerical staff—by providing, at minimum, a sheet of address labels, or preferably stamped, preaddressed envelopes, particularly if you are sending out a large number of applications to non-ERAS programs.

In conclusion, once you have successfully completed your clerkships and have carefully selected your letter writers, you can now focus on your interviews and prove that what is written on paper is actually true.

RESOURCES

Association of American Medical Colleges
www.aamc.org

Electronic Residency Application Process (ERAS)
www.aamc.org/students/eras

RESIDENT SELECTION INTERVIEWS

The interview process is time consuming and demanding, but it can also be fun and rewarding. It is the culmination of 3.5 years, or perhaps longer, of hard work in medical school. Preparation for the process will aid the applicant in succeeding. Although the interview process may be stressful, there are certain principles to follow to ensure maximal success. The residency selection interview is a job interview just as any other. The applicant must use the interview to convince the interviewers that he or she is a dedicated, hardworking, and sincere candidate who will perform to a level expected for that particular program. During the interview, it is incumbent upon the applicant to emphasize the parts of his or her application and his or her personality traits that demonstrate these facts. The interview is the time for the applicant to sell him- or herself in a genuine and honest manner. He or she must remember, however, that the interview is a two-way process. The program will try to obtain as much information about his or her as they can during this process. The interview is the time for the applicant to ask any questions that he or she may have regarding a particular program with respect to the academic, clinical, and research programs offered.

In general, interview invitations are extended beginning in early November following the submission of the dean's or medical student performance evaluation (MSPE) letter, all the way through the end of February and prior to the match in March. It is incumbent upon the applicant to respond as quickly as possible to the particular program as soon as he or she knows whether he or she wishes to accept an interview offer. If possible, the applicant should try to plan trips in order to maximize the number of interviews at one time. If programs offer several interview dates, obviously the applicant should maximize efficiency by selecting dates that maximize the number of interviews that can be accepted. If you are not going to accept a program's invitation, let them know early. This will enable them to invite other applicants to your spot. If you need to cancel a scheduled interview because of travel problems or because there is another program you would like to see, let the program know as early as possible as well. It is extremely poor form to be a no-show for an interview. This conduct may negatively affect future applicants from your medical school.

Kenneth A. Egol, MD

L. M. Jazrawi, K. A. Egol, & J. D. Zuckerman.
Orthopedic Residency & Fellowship: A Guide to Success (pp. 37-40)
© 2010 Taylor & Francis Group.

Chapter 6

Make a point to interview at your home institution's program, even if you are not interested in matching into its residency program. Use your adviser and faculty of your home institution as sources of information about possible programs. If an option is given regarding dates of interview, try to interview later in the process. Plan your day carefully. Make sure hotel, flight, and car rental reservations are made far in advance. Find out if the program where you are interviewing can help make travel arrangements at discounted rates. Make sure you know exactly how to get to the interview site on the day of the interview, and leave extra time for potential problems such as delayed hotel checkout, heavy traffic, getting lost, or other unanticipated delays. Arrive no later than 30 minutes earlier than the requested time. It is much easier to spend the rest of the time preparing for the day's events by relaxing and reading the newspaper.

DRESS/GROOMING

This is an area where you do not want to stand out. Conservative dress is the smart choice. Men should wear a dark-colored suit. Gray or blue are the best choices. Shirts should be solid white, light blue, or an off-white color. They should also be long sleeved with a conservative necktie. Be sure your suit is clean and pressed and free of stains and wrinkles. When traveling, bring a backup. Accidents happen. Remember to pack neatly. Wear dress shoes that are appropriately polished and clean. Dark socks are recommended. Be well groomed. Short neat hair is best as well as neatly shaven beards and mustaches. Jewelry should be avoided except for a watch and wedding band. Earrings, nose rings, eyebrow rings, and tongue rings do not look professional and should be removed.

For women, a suit is the best choice as well; either a skirt suit or a pantsuit without a tie is appropriate as long as it has a professional look. Skirts should be of appropriate length. Suits should be a dark, classic color such as blue, black, or gray. The same rules apply to women regarding the condition of the dress. Shoes should be conservative. Pumps or low heels that are not difficult to walk in are recommended. Shoes should be polished and clean. Women's hair should be neat, clean, and conservatively cut. Makeup should be applied neatly and not too heavily. Jewelry and accessories should be simple and conservative.

When you arrive, remember that the interview process starts as soon as you walk through the door. Always be courteous and respectful to secretaries and residency coordinators, both in person and over the phone. These people play an important role in the process and often provide feedback to the program director regarding the applicant's demeanor behind the scenes. Treat everyone as if they were making the decision to accept you. During most interviews, you will have time to meet fellow applicants and current residents of the program. This is an important time to obtain as much information as you can about the residency program. You should not give the impression that you are interested in how your free time will be spent and what social activities are available to residents.

THE INTERVIEW

Different programs have different interview styles. Some are panel interviews where you will be interviewed by several people at once. Others use a panel of interviewers with a series of one-on-one or two-on-one interviews. You will be asked certain standard questions. There are no tricks. Try not to give packaged answers. Be familiar with current events. Know what is going on in your home program, and know your own curriculum vitae (CV) inside and out. Many programs ask an ethics question. Again, there are no tricks there. Stand firm, and do not be influenced to change based on the response of the interviewer. Some programs put applicants under pressure by testing their ability to handle pressure situations. Some examples are motor skills test, reading of x-rays, and/or playing games. These are clearly tests to see how you perform under pressure. The key to success is to stay calm and answer the questions you are being asked. Take your time to answer, and remember you are not expected to be an orthopedic surgeon yet, so stay calm and focused. You should use the interview as a chance to ask questions of the interviewers to try to get some baseline information on the people involved in the interview process. Most of this is available through the Internet or through the home program's Web site. A little bit of pre-interview research can go a long way in helping the interview go smoothly. Make a list of several good questions to ask during the interview process. Try to avoid generic or trite questions.

When the interviews are done and your day is over, make sure you thank all of the residents and staff who took time to organize and participate in the interview day. Make sure you have gone on all tours and that all of your questions have been answered prior to leaving. Unless you must absolutely catch a flight and have no other options, do not leave early. Try to contemporaneously accumulate notes regarding the major issues of the program. Follow-up letters and thank-you notes may be sent to the program director as a courtesy. However, if instructed not to do so, it is not a good idea to send one anyway.

In summary, the interview process can be fun and rewarding with proper preparation and the proper attitude during the entire process. Prepare for each interview as if it were your most important one. Review your CV, and be familiar with all aspects of it. Know what questions you would like to ask. Smile, relax, be polite, and be respectful to everyone.

CHOOSING A RESIDENCY PROGRAM: THE MATCH

Upon completing the interview process, you should review the programs you visited to recall their differing characteristics. The similarities between programs far outweigh their differences and the attributes you value may be hard to identify initially. The process of selecting a residency program begins with determining your career goals and preferences. This is a daunting task made manageable when deconstructed into a discrete series of options. As each choice is made, you get closer to determining the program that is right for you. Once you have determined what you want, *The Match* helps you get it.

THE NRMP MATCH

The National Residency Match Program (NRMP) is a private, nonprofit corporation that provides an independent matching service. Established in 1952, the NRMP match provides a uniform date of appointment to graduate medical education positions, providing the opportunity for both applicants and programs to make selections only after all of the interviews have been conducted and information obtained. Without the match system, positions would be offered and accepted during the interview process, forcing both parties to make binding decisions before having explored all of their options. Since 1998, the match has been powered by the *Applicant Proposing Algorithm*. The algorithm provides an opportunity for the applicants to rank programs based solely on the applicant's interest, independent of the perceived interest from the programs. An applicant will match into the program listed highest on their list that has (1) also ranked the applicant and (2) has not filled all available positions with higher ranked candidates. A detailed description and illustrative example of the algorithm can be found at www.nrmp.org/res_match/about_res/algorithms.html. In short, consideration should only be made for your program preferences when creating the rank-order list.

Registration in the NRMP occurs in January of your graduation year and requires compliance with *Match Participation Agreement*, which outlines the enrollment requirements and contractual obligations of the match.

Daniel M. Lerman, MD and David E. Ruchelsman, MD

L. M. Jazrawi, K. A. Egol, & J. D. Zuckerman.
Orthopedic Residency & Fellowship: A Guide to Success (pp. 41-46)
© 2010 Taylor & Francis Group.

The rank-order list, submitted in February by applicants and programs, is an ordered list from the most to least desirable programs and applicants, respectively. These rank-order lists are then entered into the algorithm, which produces match results to be released on a uniform day in March at 1 pm EST. It is unlikely for a program to rank an applicant they have not interviewed, and it is ill-advised for you to list a program at which you will be unhappy as the match results are contractually binding for 1 year.

CREATING THE RANK-ORDER LIST

In order to evaluate residency programs and ultimately compile a rank-order list, it is helpful to identify specific criteria of importance to you with which to differentiate programs. Certain criteria to consider are program environment, geographic location, surgical experience, research opportunities, program size, and extent of didactic education.

There are 153 orthopedic residency programs accredited by the American College of Graduate Medical Education (ACGME). In order to receive ACGME accreditation, a program is under strict oversight and thus subject to minimum standards of education and clinical training. All programs work hard to maintain their accreditation and in doing so benefit the residents. While there is a wide range of accredited programs and many differences between them, there is no substitution for ACGME accreditation, which should be among your baseline criteria in selecting a program.

It is important to determine whether you would prefer an academic university program or a community-based program. Generally, university programs are located in more urban settings, with a larger department supporting a larger program. These programs often have more research opportunities and more extensive didactic schedules compared to community-based programs. By virtue of their research accomplishments and reputable professors, university programs often have a more notable reputation compared to community-based programs. University centers often receive referrals from the surrounding area, thereby providing the residents with greater exposure to severe and rare pathology. The reputations of academic university programs may provide an entry into preferred fellowships and serve as a foundation for a career in academic medicine.

It is typically accepted that a career transition from academic to community medicine is more easily done than the other way around. However, if you wish to practice solely clinical medicine, a community-based program offers a well-tailored experience. The community-based programs allow residents to experience local community practice and establish professional associations. Residents in community-based programs may log more cases during residency, as academic experiences are not as heavily emphasized.

Most community-based programs and some university programs lack representation of every orthopedic subspecialty. While resident training is often supplemented by away rotations at other programs, you should be aware of each program's deficits and how they are supplemented. If you have a specific subspecialty of interest, you may prefer a program well represented in that area and not have to rely on experiences outside of your program for that training. Conversely, a subspecialty may be well represented but monopolized by fellows associated with the program. You should consider the fellowships offered by each residency program and how they affect the residents' experience. It is possible for fellows to add to the residency experience or detract from it by monopolizing cases and the attendings' focus.

Fellowship training in an orthopedic subspecialty has become common among residency graduates. In evaluating any program, it is important to assess how competitive the residents are for fellowship positions, which programs they match into, and whether the residents are doing fellowships to deepen their knowledge in a particular subspecialty or to supplement insufficient surgical training during residency.

Location is a significant factor in evaluating a program, both geographically and environmentally and in terms of urban versus rural. The location of a program will dictate both where you live during residency and your local patient population. As a resident, you may want to be near friends and family or take the opportunity to explore a new region of the country. No matter where you are, the patients you see in training will invariably be from the local area. For programs in more rural settings, this may mean a more homogeneous patient population compared to the diversity of most urban centers.

While surgical and academic experiences vary widely between university and community programs, there is a wide range of experience even within these cohorts. In some programs, junior residents operate regularly. In others, operative experience is concentrated in the more senior years—"top heavy" programs. No matter how the operative experience is arranged, it is important to assess whether the residents feel comfortable with their operative skills and level of autonomy by the end of residency. Try to evaluate the resident case logs and the residents' role during surgery (primary operator or mainly observational?). Some programs brag about their resident case logs, assuming more to be better, but case logs typically fail to demonstrate the level of resident involvement during surgery. With very heavy caseloads, residents may become proficient technically while developing a deficit in knowledge or research. In reality, there is only a finite amount of time in a day/week. Consider critically how the residents in each program spend this time. Very large caseloads or extensive research may represent a deficit in another area.

Program size is another variable to consider. Orthopedic residencies vary greatly from large (>10 residents) to small (1 or 2 residents). The size of the program often reflects the size of the department and the operative volume. Larger programs frequently incorporate multiple hospitals, providing a variety of experiences (eg, a private hospital in addition to public or federal facilities). With an increase in department size and operative volume comes an increase in the number of attending physicians affiliated with a given program. Larger programs with more attending physicians offer a greater breadth of surgical and clinical experience by representing a greater range of subspecialties. Conversely, residents in smaller programs are able to spend more time with each attending, fostering deeper relationships and more personal attention.

Apart from the size of a program, it is important to determine the quality of its resources (faculty, research facilities, institutional reputation). In a surgical residency, like an apprenticeship, you learn directly from your instructors. Surgical technique, perioperative management, and patient care are all observed and disseminated through firsthand experience. Therefore, it is beneficial to work with highly trained and respected faculty. The better your instructors, the better you can become.

Part of every residency program is didactic education (lectures, journal clubs, case presentations). While the amount of time dedicated to each varies as does their scheduling, a minimum standard is established by the ACGME. Some programs have didactic sessions during weekends or evenings; others reserve a portion of time daily for a more formal educational format. Every program has a different way of creating time in the residents' busy schedule for these didactic sessions. Some programs emphasize didactics as a framework or syllabus for study, while others leave the residents to establish their own schedule for more independent learning.

For all of the above issues, there is no right or wrong answer, merely your personal preferences. Each approach has its advantages, disadvantages, proponents, and critics. You must determine what appeals to you and then find a program with those specific attributes.

Gathering information about different programs is challenging and time consuming. The most reliable source of information is your personal observation of the residents' daily routine. Because it is not possible to rotate through every program to which you applied, you must rely on other resources to make these important decisions.

Away rotations provide firsthand experience of the daily workings of a residency program, as well as the opportunity to interact with the residents and attendings. By experiencing a few different programs, you can start to identify similarities and draw comparisons to other programs with which you have only cursory exposure. In this way, away rotations provide unique insight into the specific programs and a framework with which to evaluate the other programs to which you have applied.

In most cases, the interview day is the only opportunity for you to gain personal exposure to a program and its members. While the interview day is contrived and a far departure from the daily workings of any program, it provides an opportunity to meet the residents. It is important to ask questions of the residents, but more important to observe them in their responses to you and their interactions with each other and their attendings. Observation of the residents is essential because one day that may be you—do you like what you see? Invariably, residents are complimentary of their programs. It is important to be critical of whole-hearted endorsements and appreciative of their critiques.

Due to the limited and contrived nature of the interview day, it is helpful to look toward other resources for gathering information about programs. Your orthopedic residency advisor is a good first stop for gathering information about other programs. In addition to his or her personal knowledge, he or she could direct you toward other faculty members who may have had direct experience with a program of interest.

To broaden the search for information, one can turn to the orthopedic community at large. One of the most organized and highly trafficked Web sites related to orthopedic residency is www.orthogate.org. Orthogate is an online community of medical students, residents, and attendings. The most utilized aspect of Orthogate is the forums—someone poses a question, to which others respond with a running commentary. Forum topics range widely from improving applications to thoughts on specific rotations/interviews to setting up travel arrangements. Activity on Orthogate waxes and wanes as away rotations are set up, interviews begin, and the match list is due. The broad base of participation makes the Web site useful, providing differing opinions of programs and assisting in travel arrangements. However, the Web site's contents should be judged critically with the understanding that the postings are provided by relatively anonymous self-selecting participants, resulting in an inherently biased sample of opinions. Those who are compelled to post opinions of programs, or offer advice about interviews, are the vocal minority—likely demonstrating strong feelings, positive or negative. With appreciation of this bias, Orthogate can be useful for information on programs and assistance with logistics. When receiving information about a program, it is important to consider the source, whether it is an overly enthusiastic resident or a student speaking with disdain. Everyone's advice is affected by the filter of their own personal experience.

In order to determine which programs you prefer, you must first identify your career goals and current interests. Each of the 153 ACGME-accredited orthopedic residency programs has a unique combination of the above characteristics. Any program can produce a competent orthopedist, but no program can do so without the dedication, focus, and determination of the resident. And while this chapter worked to differentiate programs based upon quantifiable criteria, in reality, a residency program is more than the sum of its parts. While it is easy to categorize programs as large or small, rural or urban, these characterizations neglect the true assets of the programs—your colleagues and faculty with whom you will be working and by whom you will be taught, instructed, and inspired.

INTERNATIONAL MEDICAL GRADUATES

There are many terms used to describe students who have attended medical school outside of the United States. The Accreditation Council for Graduate Medical Education (ACGME) uses the term *international medical graduate* (IMG) and defines the term as "a graduate from a medical school outside the United States and Canada (and not accredited by the Liaison Committee on Medical Education). IMGs may be citizens of the United States (US-IMGs) who chose to be educated elsewhere or non-citizens who are admitted to the United States by US immigration authorities (non-US–IMGs)."[1] The term *foreign medical graduate* (FMG) is often used to encompass both US and non-US citizen IMGs.

This chapter discusses specific strategies that may be beneficial to US-IMGs. While the material presented in this chapter is catered to US-IMGs, all FMGs should still refer to the other chapters in this book that provide advice for US graduates, as those discussions are also applicable and beneficial.

INTRODUCTION

Enrollment in foreign medical schools continues to rise, and the number of US-IMGs participating in the National Resident Matching Program (NRMP) has gradually increased from 2,091 in 2004 to 3,390 in 2009.[2] For those of you who are currently enrolled in a foreign medical school or are planning to attend one in the future, there are important things you need to know if you are interested in pursuing a career in orthopedic surgery. Orthopedic surgery is one of the most competitive fields in the medical profession. According to the NRMP, in 2008, 636 orthopedic surgery residency positions were available in the United States, of which 635 were filled. Of these, senior students of US allopathic schools filled 93.1%, and only 6 positions were filled by US-IMGs (0.94%).[3] The numbers have been similar in past years, and there does not seem to be any current indication that this trend is changing or that it will be easier for US-IMGs to successfully match into orthopedic surgery.

Lava Y. Patel, BA and Carl Paulino, MD

L. M. Jazrawi, K. A. Egol, & J. D. Zuckerman.
Orthopedic Residency & Fellowship: A Guide to Success (pp. 47-52)
© 2010 Taylor & Francis Group.

FIRST- AND SECOND-YEAR STUDENTS

In light of these statistics, you must devise a plan of action based on where you are in your training. If you are currently in the first 2 years of medical school, one of the most effective things you can do is to make every effort to transfer into a US medical school.

The few orthopedic attendings and residents from foreign medical schools who have successfully gone through the process have advised me numerous times throughout my training to seriously consider transferring, as it would improve my chances of matching into orthopedic surgery. Some US schools are known to take a certain number of transfer students every year. That being said, it is your responsibility to determine which US schools allow this and their individual transfer policies. You should find out which schools have accepted transfer applicants from your current school and whether there are any relationships between your current school and any particular US school. Some US schools may require you to repeat a semester or an entire year, but in the long run it will be worth it. While you are exploring your options, your main goal is to be at the top of your class academically at all times, and certainly by the time the application season begins. It cannot be stressed enough that maintaining academic excellence is critical at all times throughout your medical school training.

THIRD- AND FOURTH-YEAR STUDENTS

If you are currently in your third or fourth years of rotations, there are other options available to you. Transferring to a US medical school may still be an option. Again, look into which schools are US-IMG friendly when it comes to accepting transfer students. This may be your last opportunity to transfer into a US school. Even though you are 3 years into your training and may be required to repeat some or all of your clinical rotations, we cannot overstate how much easier the residency application process will be if you are enrolled in a US school.

Taking a year off between your third and fourth years of school to get involved with research is another potential option that may help strengthen your application. Some institutions offer a 1-year research fellowship/internship position for students during these years. These programs are usually at an academic institution where research is of great importance. For more information about research grants and positions, please refer to the section regarding research in Chapter 2.

Away/Audition Electives

As a fourth-year student, you want to maximize the number of rotations you do without burning yourself out. The more audition electives you do, the better your chances of being invited back for an interview. Many programs will offer an interview to students who have rotated with them and have done a good job, so use this time to make a positive impression. Perhaps more important than how many rotations you do is *where* you do your orthopedic surgery electives. There are programs that are more receptive to eventually matching US-IMGs than others. To find out which programs are available, the best thing to do is to speak with your student advisor and to other students in your school who have already completed their orthopedic surgery elective at certain hospitals.

After doing some research and asking around, create a list of 4 to 5 programs at which you want to rotate. Rank the hospitals in terms of your preference, how FMG friendly they are, etc. It may be in your best interest to schedule a rotation at your first choice last. This can be beneficial for many reasons. First, by having done a few electives, you will be familiar with how a typical orthopedic rotation works. You will have seen the common clinical problems encountered and will have scrubbed into many surgical cases. Once you get to your top-ranked program, you should be at the top of your game.

That being said, be careful not to burn yourself out and schedule 4 to 5 orthopedic electives back to back. By the time you rotate at your first choice, you will be exhausted. A better approach may be to schedule electives so that you do 2 months on, a few weeks off, then 2 months on. For example, I personally scheduled 2 electives for the months of July and August then took 2 weeks off in September. During these 2 weeks, I was able to concentrate on preparing and submitting all of my application materials and had some down time. From mid-September to the beginning of November, I had completed 2 more electives. At the beginning of November, I still had the option of doing yet another orthopedic elective. For those of you who still have the energy to do another, it may be a good idea, again to give yourself more options.

No matter what rotation you are on, keep in mind that you must work harder than any of the US senior students rotating with you. By no means should you ever be perceived as being lazy, as that will ultimately get back to the people who make decisions about your application. Work closely with your chief residents and do not underestimate the power of their opinions; they do matter. Chief residents can be helpful advocates or just another obstacle, depending on your performance. If you are one of those candidates who is "on the fence" in the minds of the selection committee, any negative comments from the chiefs may be the deal breaker for the program. Besides working with the chief resident, try to get exposed to the chairperson as much as possible. This will give the chairperson an opportunity to put a face to the name when reviewing your application and will also allow you the opportunity to shine in front of him or her. Get to know the residency coordinator, and do not ever annoy or irritate that person as he or she is the one who handles all of your correspondence with the program and can make sure the process goes through smoothly and in a timely fashion.

APPLYING TO ORTHOPEDIC PROGRAMS

For fourth-year students who are in the midst of applying to programs or even for third-year students who will soon be in the same situation, it is important to know the kinds of orthopedic programs available. Specifically, there are two types of programs: community programs and academic programs. The academic programs are affiliated with certain medical schools and tend to have a number of affiliated hospitals at which you would potentially work. These programs tend to be larger and offer more first-year positions. The community-based programs are smaller in size, affiliation, and number of available positions. Some students and residents believe that it may be easier for US-IMGs to successfully match at community programs over the academic programs. Whether this is true cannot be stated with certainty, but it is something you should consider when applying.

Another important consideration is the number of programs to which you should apply. Applying to a wide variety and large number of programs will likely increase your chances of being invited for an interview (but by no means will it guarantee an interview). As a US-IMG, you should keep in mind that you are fighting a harder battle than your US-school counterparts and may need to make concessions in the type of program you are willing to accept. This may mean going to a US state to which you have never been or to a smaller program than you desired, or even to a program where you will have to do an additional research year during your residency. However, in the end, your goal of becoming a certified orthopedic surgeon will be realized.

RESOURCES

A wide range of resources are available to medical students that provide advice and guidance on how to excel during rotations, how to plan electives, and how to successfully navigate the entire residency application process itself. Web sites such as www.orthogate.org are valuable tools that give you an opportunity to connect to and speak with residents and attendings in the orthopedic field in an online forum; www.valuemd.com is another online forum-based Web site that is specifically designed for foreign medical graduates and can be very helpful in answering a wide variety of questions you may have.

UNITED STATES MEDICAL LICENSING EXAMINATION

USMLE Step 1 and Step 2 Clinical Knowledge

USMLE Step 1 and Step 2 Clinical Knowledge (CK) exam scores are one of the few credentials consistently required of all applicants, domestic and foreign. These scores are among the only measures used to compare the US-IMG on the same level/standard as any US graduate. Accordingly, you must use this to your advantage and maximize your performance on these two crucial exams.

Keep in mind that US graduates who perform well on the USMLE Step 1 often delay taking the Step 2 CK exam until after they have submitted their primary applications. As a US-IMG, you may not be able to do this either because of your medical school's policy or because you may need to take and perform strongly on the Step 2 in order to strengthen your residency application prior to submitting it. No matter what, it is advisable to take the Step 2 CK exam before applying. Many program directors will not even look at an IMG's application unless it has both Step 1 and 2 CK scores. You should be well aware of your school's policy and should schedule the exams appropriately.

Every year, the NRMP publishes data on matching outcomes, which include applicants' USMLE Step scores.[4] Tables and figures illustrating the USMLE Step scores of all US Allopathic seniors and independent applicants who successfully matched are available at www.nrmp.org/data/chartingoutcomes2009v3.pdf. The "Independent Applicants" group includes all IMG's but also osteopathic students, and previous US Allopathic graduates. However, it should still give you an idea of where you stand.

USMLE Step 2 Clinical Skills

The USMLE Step 2 Clinical Skills (CS) exam is intended to evaluate one's clinical skills using clinical encounters with live patients. It is an 8-hour exam that requires you to evaluate 12 patients with common medical complaints. You will be given a total of 25 minutes per patient, with 15 minutes allotted for taking a history and physical exam and 10 minutes for writing a patient note summarizing your history, physical findings, differential diagnosis, and patient work-up.

IMGs are most likely to fail this exam because of poor communication/interpersonal skills.[5] Proper preparation may take anywhere from 1 week to a couple of months. Start early on in your preparation to determine how much time you will need to ensure you pass on the first try. There are several study aids available to help you prepare for this exam, and perhaps the most commonly used is a book titled *First Aid for the USMLE Step 2 CS*, written by Tao Le and Vikas Bhushan.[5] It is also recommended that you study with a partner, preferably a medical student, so that you can practice history taking and the physical exam on one another.

The Step 2 CS exam is also one that may be mandatory for you to complete prior to applying. Program directors need to know that foreign applicants are clinically competent. Do not risk having your application delayed or not even considered because of missing test scores. In addition to making you look irresponsible, and therefore not putting your best foot forward, it can also jeopardize your chances of being timely and fully considered for a position.

BE PREPARED IF YOU DON'T MATCH

It is important for US-IMGs to be aware of and realistic about their chances of successfully matching into an orthopedic residency program. If you do not match the first time you apply, here are some options you may consider:

- ✓ Do a preliminary year of general surgery at the hospital at which you would potentially like to match into orthopedics.
- ✓ Become an orthopedic house officer/house staff at the hospital at which you would like to match.
- ✓ Conduct a year of research with the orthopedics department either at the hospital where you would like to match or at a large institution alongside an influential attending or national figure in the field.
- ✓ Apply for a categorical general surgery position. After completing your general surgery residency, you can apply for a reconstructive plastic/hand surgery fellowship. This is another possible route to take if you would like to practice hand surgery.
- ✓ Consider other fields that involve the musculoskeletal system—specialties such as rheumatology, physical medicine and rehabilitation, or sports medicine.
- ✓ Re-evaluate what you want out of your professional career, and see if there may be another specialty out there for you where you could be just as happy and fulfilled.

CONCLUSION

Matching into a competitive residency such as orthopedic surgery is not an easy task, but do not be discouraged because it has happened in the past and will continue to happen in the future. The best thing you can do is to understand the entire process and present yourself in the best way possible. Keep in mind at all times that in this very competitive environment, program directors are looking for reasons not to take you, and it is your job to give them reasons for just the opposite. We hope the suggestions made in this chapter continue to give you hope and encouragement in pursuing a career in orthopedic surgery.

REFERENCES

1. Accreditation Council for Graduate Medical Education. Glossary of terms. September 18, 2009. Available at: http://acgme.org/acWebsite/about/ab_ACGMEglossary.pdf. Accessed November 17, 2009.
2. National Resident Matching Program. Advanced Data Tables: 2009 Main Residency Match. 2008. Available at: http://www.nrmp.org/data/advancedatatables2009.pdf. Accessed November 17, 2009.
3. National Resident Matching Program. Advanced Data Tables: 2008 Main Residency Match. 2008. Available at: http://www.nrmp.org/data/advancedatatables2008.pdf. Accessed November 17, 2009.
4. National Resident Matching Program. Charting Outcomes in the Match: Characteristics of Applicants Who Matched to Their Preferred Specialty in the 2009 NRMP Main Residency Match. 3rd ed. 2009. Available at: http://www.nrmp.org/data/chartingoutcomes2009v3.pdf. Accessed November 17, 2009.
5. Le T, Bhushan V. *First Aid for the USMLE Step 2 CS*. 3rd ed. New York, NY: McGraw-Hill Medical; 2009.

WHAT TO DO IF YOU DON'T MATCH

As Match Day approaches, if you are one of the medical students who received early notification that you did not match, it will probably be the first time in your life that you were unable to achieve the goal you had established for yourself. You will be overcome by so many emotions—disappointment, anger, sorrow—and will ask, "How did this happen?" and "Why did this happen to me?" Although this may seem like the darkest time in your life, it is a time to take a step back and try, as much as possible, to evaluate the situation in which you find yourself. Only in this way can you take the steps necessary to increase your chances of successfully achieving your goals.

Although there may be a few unfilled positions available each year, the chance of obtaining one of these positions in the "scramble" is small. Nonetheless, you should pursue each one immediately. Submit your application material, including all letters of recommendation to each program with a position(s) available. You should do this even if it is a program you had previously applied to (or even interviewed at). Although the chances are admittedly small, this is a necessary first step when you have not successfully matched. If you are successful in obtaining one of these positions, you can feel great relief and can move on to Section II of this book. The remainder of this chapter will focus on strategies to use when you have not been successful in securing a position.

The first step is to realistically assess your application "package"; specifically, to identify areas of weakness. Potential areas of weakness can include the following:

- ✔ Academic performance
- ✔ Letters of recommendation
- ✔ Application strategy
- ✔ Interviewing

Careful assessment of these different factors will lead you to 1 of 4 options for moving forward:

Joseph D. Zuckerman, MD

L. M. Jazrawi, K. A. Egol, & J. D. Zuckerman.
Orthopedic Residency & Fellowship: A Guide to Success (pp. 53-60)
© 2010 Taylor & Francis Group.

1. Identify and secure a preliminary first post-graduate year (PGY-1) position, graduate from medical school as scheduled, and plan on reapplying the following year.

2. Graduate from medical school as scheduled and begin a 1- to 2-year research fellowship in orthopedic surgery to strengthen your application.

3. Delay your graduation from medical school and complete 1 year of full-time orthopedic research to further strengthen your application.

4. Identify a PGY-1 position, graduate from medical school as scheduled, and decide to pursue residency training in an area other than orthopedic surgery.

The key is to match the assessment of your application package with 1 of the 4 options listed. To do this will require a careful assessment of your qualifications to determine your potential to match when you reapply.

ACADEMIC PERFORMANCE

Academic performance is the most important component of your application. Because few medical schools provide specific information concerning class rank, academic performance is generally based upon United States Medical Licensing Examination (USMLE) Step 1 scores (because most students have not taken USMLE Step 2 by the time the application is submitted) and honors grades during the pre-clinical years and particularly for clinical clerkships. Of course, selection for membership in the Alpha Omega Alpha (AΩA) Honor Society is another important variable, but it would be very uncommon for an AΩA student to not match. If this did occur, it would require a careful evaluation of interviewing techniques and application strategy. The dean's letter of recommendation for some schools provides an assessment of the applicant's performance relative to the rest of the class, but this tends to be quite variable from school to school and will not be known to the applicant. Let's first discuss USMLE Step 1.

The average USMLE Step 1 score is approximately 220. A score below 200 will be very difficult to overcome and may, in and of itself, be the primary reason for not matching. With this score, particularly in the absence of honors for required third year clinical clerkships, anyone reviewing the application will note a significant academic deficiency. In this situation, there is probably some value in using USMLE Step 2 to overcome a low Step 1 score. A very high score on USMLE Step 2 may have a very positive impact. However, this will vary from program to program, depending on the emphasis that each program places on Step 1 versus Step 2. If you have not already taken Step 2 at the time of the Match, then all efforts should be focused on the Step 2 exam in an effort to make it a strength of your application and limit the negative impact of a poor Step 1 score.

The clerkship grades are also determined by this time, and little, if any, action can be taken to modify their impact. If you have had some high pass or honors grades, particularly during third-year clerkships, this will be considered a strength and is a reason to reapply. Honors grades in the fourth year are less significant but do have some value and once again would strengthen your reapplication.

If your Step 1 score was above average, then it will be important to look for other areas that may have been limiting your application. This could be grades on clinical clerkships, which, unfortunately, cannot be improved. However, the problem may frequently be in another area (ie, letters of recommendation, interviewing, and application strategy), which will be discussed.

The most important aspect in the evaluation of academic performance is a realistic assessment of whether it is an insurmountable limitation. If you feel this is the case, then it would be best to consider pursuing other areas of residency training. However, if you feel that your academic performance does not have glaring weaknesses but may not have been "at a high enough level," then the goal should be to enhance your credentials and reapply. As noted, this can be accomplished in part by an outstanding score on USMLE Step 2. However, it is my opinion that it is most effectively accomplished by devoting at least 1 year to orthopedic research in an effort to separate yourself from the remainder of the applicant pool. I think this is a better approach than entering a PGY-1 preliminary position in which your rotations generally do not allow significant exposure to orthopedic surgery and, even more importantly, orthopedic faculty who would be willing to support your application. This is particularly true because you will be reapplying for residency training after only 2 months of the PGY-1 year. It is unlikely that during this time you would be able to obtain meaningful new letters of recommendation that would strengthen your application.

I cannot overemphasize the importance of a careful and objective evaluation of your academic qualifications in order to determine how to proceed. This is best accomplished with the assistance of a person knowledgeable in the area. This could be your faculty advisor, the orthopedic residency program director at your school, or a member of the dean's office, preferably the one who prepared your dean's letter. As difficult as this may be, it is the most critical step in determining how to proceed and, specifically, whether reapplying is in your best interest.

I would emphasize that in all the meetings I have had with medical students who have not matched, there have been only one or two instances in which my recommendation was not to reapply. Significant academic deficiencies are usually factored into the decision making of which residency to pursue. Given the competitive nature of the orthopedic surgery Match, students with a deficient academic performance will most often select a different specialty area. For the vast majority of students who do not successfully match, the decision will be to reapply and present the strongest "application package" possible.

LETTERS OF RECOMMENDATION

The impact of your letters of recommendation is difficult to assess since the content is not known to each applicant because you have "waived your right to review the letter." Nonetheless, it is essential to completely evaluate the letters of recommendation you have submitted previously, specifically to determine whether these same individuals should be asked to do so again.

The dean's letter is a somewhat special circumstance. When you reapply, the dean's letter will be updated and resubmitted. It is important to meet with the dean who is responsible for preparing the letter. The new letter will be enhanced by additional information that will include the results of your fourth-year clerkships (which can be very positive if you did well), the results of USMLE Step 2, and information about your additional activities following the completion of your fourth year. This may be a description of the research program you decided to pursue for a year or your decision to complete a PGY-1 year. It is very important to meet with the dean and use this as an opportunity to have an impact on the revised letter that will be prepared.

Your other letters of recommendation should be evaluated very carefully. You should consider who prepared your letters previously and then think about the additional group of faculty members with whom you have worked during your fourth-year clerkships.

The goal is to ask those faculty members who can prepare the strongest possible letter for you. Although it is difficult to determine what a faculty member will write, it is essential to have a reasonable "sense" so you can choose wisely. The most ideal letter is one that describes you as "the best medical student I have worked with in 5 years" or something comparable. Letters like this are best provided by faculty members who know you well, and this should be an overriding factor in your selection.

Of course, letters of recommendation should be sought from faculty members with whom you work following completion of your fourth year, whether as part of a research year(s) or as part of a PGY-1 year. The same principles apply—choose wisely and focus on those faculty members who can recommend you in the strongest possible way.

APPLICATION STRATEGY

If you are unsuccessful in your Match efforts, it is important to evaluate your application strategy to determine what changes should be made. Application strategy refers to the number and types of programs you apply to; it does not relate to the content of your application, which has been discussed previously.

The goal of your application strategy is to be invited for as many interviews as possible. The only programs that will consider you as a candidate are the ones where you have interviewed. The goal of your application strategy should be to have at least 10 interviews. If you accomplished this and did not match, then you should focus on 2 areas when reapplying:

1. A careful evaluation of your interview techniques for potential problems—this will be discussed in the next section

2. Designing an application strategy that will result in at least 10 interviews, and preferably more, to maximize your chance of matching

If you have interviewed at fewer than 10 programs, then your primary focus in reapplying should be to develop an application strategy that increases the number of interview invitations. The question to be considered is why you did not receive at least 10 interviews. Was this because of academic deficiencies in your application, along the lines of the issues discussed earlier in this chapter? Or, was it because you applied to too few programs? It is hard to imagine any applicant not applying to at least 30 programs based upon the competitive nature of the orthopedic Match. In general, as your concerns about the academic strength of your application increase, so should the number of applications submitted. When reapplying, it is important to consider both the number of programs you apply to as well as the specific programs you select. The number of programs you apply to should increase, and, in most cases, this will include at least 50 programs. The programs you select should reflect a realistic assessment of your qualifications, combined with your experiences when you applied previously (where did you interview, where did you complete rotations, feedback from your own faculty members). It is probably not realistic to apply to the most competitive programs unless you feel your "reapplication package" has improved significantly. As for geography and program size, these are factors that you can consider. However, the most important question to ask yourself is, "What is more important—matching to *any* program or living in a specific geographic area or training in a program of a specific size?" The answers to these questions should invariably be that matching is the most important, regardless of program location or program size. Of course, there may be extenuating family or personal issues that would change this approach, which is an issue that each individual will need to assess.

In general, the application strategy when reapplying should be to obtain as many interviews as possible. To do so will require applying to a large number of programs depending upon the competitiveness of your application. Although the cost of applying to programs increases as the number of applications increases, this expense will be relatively small. The cost of interviews is more significant, but once again, a successful Match is more likely to occur as the number of interviews increases. The expense involved in interviewing is a necessary component of successfully matching to an orthopedic program.

INTERVIEWING

For many programs, including ours, the interview is a very important component of the application process. We have always told our applicants that once you are selected for an interview, you are essentially on "equal footing" with all of the other applicants regardless of academic performance or where you attend medical school. Therefore, the interview can be expected to be the primary factor in determining your rank on a program's Match list.

There are 2 issues to consider related to interviewing: quantity and quality. If you interviewed at only 3 programs and did not match, then clearly the goal will be to increase the number of interviews obtained when you reapply. The most important strategies to accomplish this relate to the strength of your application and the number of programs to which you apply. These factors have been discussed previously. However, if you interviewed in at least 7 or 8 programs and did not match, it is important to carefully evaluate the "quality" of your interview. In this context, it is important to ask yourself, "What is it about my interview that may have had a negative impact on my application?" This can be a difficult question to answer because it requires you to be very introspective and self-critical of your interview presentation. Interviewing is like everything else we do. It is a learned skill that improves with experience. Although some individuals may interview better than others, it is possible to improve one's interview skills with feedback and training. If you feel that your interview performance may have been problematic, it would be very helpful to obtain direct feedback from one of your interviewers. This may be most easily accomplished at your own program, possibly with the assistance of your faculty advisor. Direct, candid feedback about your interviewing skills can be difficult to obtain, but it is an important area to pursue. It has the potential to provide important information that will guide you through your future interviews. In some cases, it can be helpful to meet with professionals about interviewing techniques. The human resources department in your medical school or hospital should be able to provide information in this area.

It is also important to ask yourself whether you prepared properly for interviews. Most questions are predictable and tend to be repeated from one interview to another. Being prepared for these questions is important, but answering the questions in a way that does not appear to be "automatic" is also important. You should also evaluate your presentation during the interview. Did you dress appropriately? Did you sit properly during the interview? Did you conduct yourself in a laid-back or an overly aggressive manner? One problem I have encountered in the interview process is when applicants interview with the residents, particularly in a program where he or she may have rotated. There may be a certain level of familiarity that develops, which can compromise the interview. It is important to conduct yourself appropriately with residents as well as with faculty members you may know well. You should recognize that your presentation during interviews should be consistent and not vary significantly based upon your familiarity with the interviewer.

Overall, it is very important for you to evaluate your interview technique in preparation for reapplying. Each interview becomes that much more important, and your goal should be to make certain that your interview increases your chance of matching and does not do anything to compromise it.

FOUR OPTIONS

Of the 4 options listed previously, it can be difficult to provide definitive recommendations as to which option is best under specific circumstances. However, there are general guidelines that can be helpful.

Option 1—securing a preliminary PGY-1 position and reapplying during the PGY-1 year—may be best for individuals who feel that their application package is strong enough to successfully match and the deficiencies related more to application strategy and possibly interviewing technique. It is important to recognize that completion of the PGY-1 year will really be an extra year because all programs match into a 5-year program, which will necessitate repeating the PGY-1 year. Occasionally, a PGY-2 position may be available, but this situation is very uncommon. It has always been my opinion that this option is more limiting and, because the PGY-1 year will often be an extra year, that year is better devoted to strengthening your application. In addition, time off for interviews can usually be more easily accomplished during a research year. However, your personal situation may necessitate entering a preliminary PGY-1 year, and this is a decision that should be made on an individual basis.

Option 4—identify a PGY-1 position and decide to pursue residency training in an area other than orthopedic surgery—is obviously most appropriate for those individuals who decide that the deficiencies in their application package cannot be overcome, and it would be very unlikely that they would successfully match when reapplying, even if additional steps are taken to strengthen the application. This requires a careful and often painfully objective evaluation of your application. I would suggest that this decision be made in discussions with your faculty advisor and the Dean of Students so that all of the factors are carefully considered.

I have always considered options 2 and 3, which include completion of a research fellowship to strengthen your application, to be the most helpful in strengthening an application. The decision to complete a research fellowship is an individual one, and it is based upon personal factors as well as the availability of suitable fellowship positions. Recently, some orthopedic fellowships have required 2 years, while others are limited to 1 year. A concern inherent in options 2 or 3 is the decision of whether to delay your medical school graduation. My opinion is that it is better to reapply as a medical student rather than having graduated medical school and being in that "hiatus" between completion of medical school and the beginning of residency training. I think continuing as a fifth-year medical student changes the nature of the dean's letter in a positive way and changes how you are viewed by programs evaluating your application. I also recognize this is an individual decision and will be determined by a variety of factors. Many research fellowships do not provide sufficient financial support, and the economic burden may be problematic for many students.

Of the 4 options listed, there are clearly some specific factors that will make one option more attractive than others. In selecting the option that is best for you, it is important to devote the time needed to make a careful and informed decision. This is another reason why I believe it is best not to immediately "scramble" for a PGY-1 position. This is an important decision that requires careful thought and analysis as well as discussions with your advisors and your family, so take the amount of time needed to arrive at a decision that is best for you.

In summary, not matching to an orthopedic surgery residency program will present you with both personal and professional challenges. If this occurs, it is important to take a step back and objectively evaluate the situation and determine the best options for how to proceed. This will certainly vary from one individual to the next, but there are basic principles and approaches that should be followed. A realistic assessment of the strengths and weaknesses of your application combined with integration of personal factors will allow you to determine the best course of action. I would emphasize the importance of seeking advice from your faculty mentors and the dean's office. Like each and every problem we may face, this one will also benefit from careful analysis and strategic planning.

Section II

INTERNSHIP

Congratulations on the match! Welcome to one of the most rewarding professions in medicine. Your years of hard work and dedication have paid off, and you are now an orthopedic surgery resident. The first year of residency, also known as the first postgraduate year (PGY-1) or more affectionately as the internship, marks the beginning of the exciting and intellectually stimulating 5-year journey of the orthopedic surgery residency that every orthopedic surgeon must undertake. You were selected to be a resident physician at your program after a very long and intensive process that started the day you decided you wanted to be an orthopedic surgeon. The internship year provides you with the foundation upon which you will build to become a compassionate, knowledgeable, and technically sound orthopedic surgeon. It is very important that you continue to display the same attributes that allowed you to become a top medical student and earned you one of these highly sought-after residency positions. Although you are now an orthopedic surgery resident, you must continue to read the latest literature and work hard so that you are prepared to provide your patients with the best medical care. It is also absolutely imperative that you understand your new position on the team, the accompanying expectations, and your responsibilities. The intern year has a very steep learning curve, in which you go from being a fourth-year medical student in May to being the physician responsible for the well-being of several patients in late June or early July.

The intern year typically commences in late June with a series of orientation lectures and basic certification courses, such as the Advanced Cardiac Life Support (ACLS) course. The orientation activities also provide you with the opportunity to explore the medical center's facilities and learn the medical record system. Most importantly, it provides the opportunity to meet and interact with your co-interns. Needless to say, the intern year will be one of the most challenging, yet exciting and rewarding years of your career. This is when you start to build your knowledge base and the psychomotor skills necessary to be an excellent surgeon. This chapter will provide you with a guide on how to maximize your intern year and create good habits that will serve you well for the rest of your career.

Kirk A. Campbell, MD and Eric J. Strauss, MD

L. M. Jazrawi, K. A. Egol, & J. D. Zuckerman.
Orthopedic Residency & Fellowship: A Guide to Success (pp. 63-68)
© 2010 Taylor & Francis Group.

THE INTERN YEAR

So what does the intern year consist of? Although the exact composition of the intern year varies at different institutions, the Accreditation Council for Graduate Medical Education (ACGME) has created guidelines that allow each residency program director to create a well-rounded PGY-1 experience and also ensure some uniformity in the training provided at different programs. The typical intern year, like the one at our institution, consists of 12 rotations on various services. However, no more than 3 months may be spent on orthopedic surgery. Six months must be spent on various surgical services and may be chosen from plastic surgery, vascular surgery, general surgery, trauma surgery, or cardiothoracic surgery. Finally, the last 3 months may be selected from the following associated disciplines: emergency medicine, anesthesia, musculoskeletal imaging, or critical care. Many of you may be asking yourselves about the purpose of the non-orthopedic surgery rotations. These rotations are absolutely critical to your development as a physician, because although you will focus on musculoskeletal disorders in your practice, it is absolutely imperative that you have an understanding of the perioperative, intraoperative, and postoperative management of patients. The non-orthopedic surgery rotations allow you to build a solid knowledge base by exposing you to the acute management of trauma patients with multiple organ system injuries, management of chronic medical co-morbidities and critical care issues, soft tissue management, as well as an understanding of surgical anesthesia. These rotations allow you to develop the diagnostic skills necessary to effectively indentify potential problems and the clinical judgment to decide if your team will be able to effectively manage the patient, or if the assistance of an expert consultant is needed. These rotations are structured to allow one to develop as a physician within the system of the 6 core competencies for training physicians developed by the ACGME and will be highlighted throughout this chapter. The rotations provide you a certain level of confidence that allows you to manage stable medical problems without the help of a consultant and also the ability to stabilize a patient during an acute event before you are able to call the appropriate consultant to assist in management. Thus, the intern year allows you to gain the necessary skills to provide your patient with optimal medical care (ACGME core competency—patient care).

The intern year also provides you with the opportunity to interact with co-interns, senior residents, and faculty members from other services, which allows you to build potentially long-lasting social and professional relationships. Rotating on the non-orthopedic surgery specialties also provides you with the perfect opportunity to begin studying for the United States Medical Licensing Examination (USMLE) Step 3, which is the last part of the USMLE series that is required to obtain the medical license. Although you are not required to take this exam during the intern year, it is highly recommended, because the intern year provides you with exposure to the widest variety of medical disciplines that are tested on this 2-day exam. Furthermore, studying for this exam affords you the opportunity to review all of the concepts you learned in medical school and will allow you to become a well-rounded physician earlier in your career.

Needless to say, it is absolutely imperative that you are the consummate team player and hard worker regardless of the rotation that you are on. There is a common misconception that you only have to work hard when you are on the orthopedic surgery service. This is absolutely wrong! You should maintain a solid work ethic regardless of the rotation or department because you are always a representative of the orthopedic surgery department. Evaluations from these rotations are reviewed by your program director, and your performance during the year is monitored by your program's resident evaluation committee. Furthermore, the intern year is when you begin to build your reputation, and one never wants to be known as someone with a poor work ethic or who is difficult to work with. You are the best and the brightest, and you must demonstrate the same high-level commitment to every rotation.

THE TEAM AND YOUR RESPONSIBILITY

Residency training consists of a hierarchical structure in which the attending physician is the highest person in the command chain. The chief resident or another senior resident is the captain of the team, which may also consist of junior residents and you, the intern. It is very important to respect this chain of command, but also never to be intimidated by it. The intern is generally the person who is most involved in the fine details of patient care. There is also a larger team of nurses, social workers, and ancillary staff who help to facilitate the highest level of medical care for your patients (ACGME core competency—professionalism). The intern will often be the first person contacted about patient care issues. The intern is often involved in the full spectrum of patient care from the patient's admission straight through to discharge and the appropriate outpatient follow-up (ACGME core competency—practice-based learning). It is very important to be professional and conscientious in all of your interactions with the nurses and ancillary staff, especially when they contact you while you are extremely busy trying to take care of other issues. It is very important to prioritize all of your tasks, address all of the life-threatening issues—such as quickly seeing a patient with chest pain or shortness of breath—first, and then work your way down to less important things—such as to changing a patient's diet order or ordering acetaminophen (Tylenol).

You should never be afraid to ask for help. It is expected that you will require assistance in managing patients. However, before you request assistance, it is absolutely necessary that you gather all of the pertinent information so that you are able to accurately communicate it to your senior resident. For example, if you are paged in the middle of an extremely busy night and are informed that one of your patients has a fever, you must be able to quickly develop a differential diagnosis list that will allow you to ask the nurse appropriate questions and determine the acuity of the situation. These questions will also allow you to prioritize the situation and determine the order in which you will go and evaluate the patient. It is very important to always do the proper work-up and avoid shortcuts, which can lead to catastrophic outcomes. So if a patient needs to be cultured or taken to another part of the hospital for further studies, it is your duty to perform the necessary test.

Additionally, you should always remember that you are not alone, and you should inform your senior residents of any acute changes in a patient's status. The process of developing a differential diagnosis list and thoroughly evaluating the patient will allow you to convey this information to your senior resident. You should also constantly contemplate potential questions that a consultant or a more senior member of your team may have if you need to ask them for help. You should never try to be a "hero" and manage challenging situations by yourself. Regardless of how thorough you were in evaluating a sick patient, a more experienced person will inevitably ask a question about the patient that you did not consider and may not have the information (ACGME core competency—systems-based practice). This is expected at your level of training and should be used as a learning experience to build your fund of knowledge. Honesty is absolutely essential, because lying about something you did not do or making up lab values can negatively affect a patient by making a dire situation look benign.

HOW TO BE A GOOD INTERN

As was alluded to in the previous section, a good intern is the consummate team player. The ideal intern is a conscientious and compassionate person who is able to stay organized, efficiently manage patients, and effectively communicate with other members of the team (ACGME core competency—interpersonal and communication skills). Unfortunately, becoming a good intern is a slow process that everyone must go through. This process starts on the first day of your residency training and is continually refined throughout the year. One of the most important things to learn is how to prioritize your tasks, because invariably you will be asked to complete a very long list of things. Organizing these tasks will allow you to efficiently complete them. Note that, regardless of how hard you work to complete all of your assigned tasks, there will be some tasks that you are unable to finish for a variety of reasons. Some senior residents may be insensitive to this and may provide you with the notorious "beat down," in which they tell you something that always starts off with the proverbial "when I was an intern..." You should never take these outbursts personally, because no matter how hard you try, you will never satisfy everyone. However, you should always sincerely try to complete your tasks and ask for help when you realize everything may not get done.

Another way to be a good intern is to be proactive and offer your assistance to the other members of your team, especially the junior residents. Helping a junior resident see consults is a very high-yield educational experience because it provides you with exposure to a wide variety of injuries and the management challenges they entail. Shadowing the more senior residents in the free time you have after you have completed all of your tasks demonstrates to them your interest in learning new things. Showing an interest in learning will lead to the more senior residents seeking you out to teach you whenever they have an interesting case or reduction. If you are already comfortable with a procedure, you should invite one of your co-interns along so that he or she may also benefit from the teaching session with the senior resident. It is no secret that most residents love to teach their more junior peers how to manage patients, reduce fractures, and apply splints. Some of the other skills that you should try to acquire during your internship include evaluating a patient with a musculoskeletal injury and understanding the role that the mechanism of injury plays. Furthermore, learning how to perform a good physical exam, aspirating joints, and inserting traction pins will be a huge asset. Learning the proper imaging studies and views to order, as well as how to accurately read the films, are other essential skills that your more senior residents can teach you. Performing a thorough physical exam and obtaining the appropriate films will provide you with a majority of diagnoses. You should never be lazy and accept a substandard view, because this may lead to the mismanagement of the patient's injuries. These activities will give you a boost going into your second year, when you may be asked to be the consult resident for your service.

HOW TO BUILD A GOOD KNOWLEDGE BASE

The intern year marks a major transition point in both your social and professional life. It marks perhaps the first time in your life when there is no teacher or professor to tell you what to expect on the prescheduled exam. You have made it this far into your career by preparing for exams; however, to be a successful orthopedic surgeon, you must now transition from studying or cramming for exams to truly learning principles and applying them to each unique patient encounter. Daily patient care activities provide you with multiple pop quizzes and major exams; therefore, it is imperative that you are thoroughly prepared. To facilitate your development into a lifelong learner, a well-respected member of my department recommends that "you read every single day...even on vacation." Reading is the only way that you will be able to build your knowledge base (ACGME core competency—medical knowledge).

A common intern complaint is that there is no time to read. However, if you manage your time appropriately, the intern year affords a tremendous opportunity to start building a solid foundation that will serve you well throughout your residency. The time constraints will continue to increase as you progress through residency, so implementing solid study habits now will allow you to better manage your time. Anatomy is by far the most important topic for an intern to read. Having a mastery of musculoskeletal anatomy will serve you well the rest of your career because the practice of orthopedics is essentially applied anatomy. *Netter's Concise Atlas of Orthopaedic Anatomy* by Thompson and *Surgical Exposures in Orthopaedics: The Anatomic Approach* by Hoppenfeld and DeBoer are 2 excellent resources to learn musculoskeletal anatomy. A good strategy to employ is to carry a pocket-sized orthopedics handbook—such as the *Handbook of Fractures* or the *Manual of Orthopaedics*—or one of the excellent review articles from *Journal of the American Academy of Orthopaedic Surgeons* in your white coat. This will allow you to quickly read it when you find yourself with some down time in the hospital. Reading about the consults you see with senior residents or about your clinic patient's condition is a good way to augment these experiences. It is important to note that you are not expected to become an expert this year, but this reading will familiarize you with the terminology and key concepts that you need to know during the PGY-2 year and beyond. Preparing for conferences and the rare operating room case will also allow you to get the maximum educational value from these activities and will allow you to ask intelligent questions.

The Orthopaedic In-Training Exam (OITE) is a standardized exam that all orthopedic surgery residents across the country take in the fall. This exam allows residents to assess their fund of knowledge, while also providing information to chart their progress against their peers at the same level of training. Although interns may not be required to take this exam, developing a structured reading schedule will facilitate studying for this exam. Furthermore, if your program does not require you to take the exam as an intern, then reading now will provide you with an edge in your studying. The Recommended Reading section in this chapter provides a very limited sampling of some of the study resources available.

MAINTAINING BALANCE IN YOUR LIFE

One of the greatest challenges you will face as an intern is how to make time for yourself. As physicians, we have mastered the art of taking care of others, but at times we may forget to take care of ourselves. Finding the right balance between your life inside and outside of the hospital is absolutely essential for reducing some of the inherent stress of residency training. Making time for family and friends should be placed on your priority list. Although your family will need to have a certain level of understanding about the sometimes unpredictable nature of orthopedics, you should always make time in your schedule to spend with your loved ones. Developing or continuing healthy eating habits and partaking in cardiovascular exercise will help to alleviate some of the stresses of the intern year. Furthermore, you should try to continue to enjoy the things you did in medical school to relax as time permits.

RULES OF HOW TO BE A SUCCESSFUL INTERN

The following rules will not only allow you to survive the intern year, but will also allow you to excel and enjoy the year.

- ✓ Always work hard.
- ✓ Be a team player.
- ✓ Never take short cuts with patient care. Always do the full work-up.
- ✓ Be honest.
- ✓ Always be early (to rounds, conference, etc).
- ✓ Read every single day to build your knowledge base.
- ✓ Be professional.
- ✓ Respect the chain of command.
- ✓ Always provide patients with the best medical care.
- ✓ Create a balance between work and your personal life.
- ✓ Be able to take constructive criticism and ignore mean-spirited people who mistreat you.
- ✓ Always be available to help.
- ✓ Shadow senior residents to learn procedures and physical exam techniques.
- ✓ Follow work hour guidelines.
- ✓ Enjoy the year!

RECOMMENDED READING

Browner B, Levine A, Jupiter J, Trafton P, Krettek C. *Skeletal Trauma: Basic Science, Management, and Reconstruction*. 4th ed. Philadelphia, PA: Saunders; 2008.

Canale ST, Beaty JH. *Campbell's Operative Orthopaedics*. 11th ed. Philadelphia, PA: Mosby Elsevier; 2008.

Hoppenfeld S. *Physical Exam of the Spine and Extremities*. Upper Saddle River, NJ: Prentice Hall; 1976.

Hoppenfeld S, DeBoer P. *Surgical Exposures in Orthopaedics: The Anatomic Approach*. 3rd ed. Philadelphia, PA: Lippincott Williams & Wilkins; 2003.

Journal of the American Academy of Orthopaedic Surgeons. Published monthly by the American Academy of Orthopaedic Surgeons, Rosemont, IL. Available at: www.jaaos.org.

Koval KJ, Zuckerman JD. *Handbook of Fractures*. 3rd ed. Philadelphia, PA: Lippincott Williams & Wilkins; 2006.

Lieberman JR. *AAOS Comprehensive Orthopaedic Review*. Rosemont, IL: American Academy of Orthopedic Surgeons; 2009.

Miller MD. *Review of Orthopaedics*. 5th ed. Philadelphia, PA: Saunders; 2008.

Rockwood CA, Green DP. *Rockwood and Green's Fractures in Adults*. 6th ed. Philadelphia, PA: Lippincott Williams & Wilkins; 2006.

Swiontkowski M, Stovitz SD. *Manual of Orthopaedics*. 6th ed. Philadelphia, PA: Lippincott Williams & Wilkins; 2006.

Thompson J. *Netter's Concise Atlas of Orthopaedic Anatomy*. Teterboro, NJ: Icon Learning Systems; 2002.

RESIDENCY SURVIVAL SKILLS: KEYS TO SUCCESS

After a year as a surgical intern learning how to take care of preoperative and postoperative patients and figuring out how to be effective and efficient in the hospital setting, you are finally ready to develop the skills necessary to become an orthopedic surgeon. You are now an orthopedic surgery resident, and you have the next 4 years (for now) to learn as much as you can about musculoskeletal pathology and its operative management. The path to this ultimate goal is long and at times trying, but remember that this will be the basis for the rest of your professional career.

Being a successful orthopedic resident requires a great deal of dedication and responsibility. The following rules of residency/survival skills/keys to success will serve you well—if you are able to adhere to them, you will be a resident that the attending staff and your peers know they can depend on and one whom your junior residents will look up to.

RULE #1: TREAT YOUR FELLOW RESIDENTS AS YOU WOULD EXPECT TO BE TREATED

This may seem simple or common sense but it needs to be emphasized. Your ability to work well within your team and with the other residents in your program will become evident relatively quickly in your training. The goal is to be a role model for everyone around you. A resident who is always willing to help out his or her peers, whether it is covering a night of call when a conflict arises or scrubbing an extra case when coverage is short, is much more pleasant to work with than one who is lazy, is undependable, or has the reputation of "dumping" on their classmates or juniors. In the hospital working environment, all things are noticed, and your goal should be to have the respect of your peers. Four years of training is a long haul, and having a good working relationship with your fellow residents is paramount to an enjoyable experience.

Eric J. Strauss, MD and David E. Ruchelsman, MD

L. M. Jazrawi, K. A. Egol, & J. D. Zuckerman.
Orthopedic Residency & Fellowship: A Guide to Success (pp. 69-74)
© 2010 Taylor & Francis Group

RULE #2: RECOGNIZE THE HIERARCHY ON YOUR SERVICE AND WITHIN THE RESIDENCY PROGRAM

Understanding the structure of your team will help define whom you are responsible to and whom you are responsible for. Having a well-defined role will enable you to make the most of the experience and will provide you with the opportunity to learn from your seniors while at the same time to educate your juniors. Respecting the hierarchy will also enable you to avoid many problems if and when they arise. The "bump it up" mentality will without fail keep you out of trouble and, most times, lead to a solution for even the most complicated situation, whether it be with patient care or administrative red tape.

RULE #3: KNOW WHERE YOU SHOULD BE AND WHEN YOU NEED TO BE THERE

Being on time for rounds, clinic, and operative cases is of paramount importance. It is a direct reflection of your level of dedication and responsibility. Showing up at 6:30 am on the dot for 6:30 am rounds means you are 10 minutes late. Attendings tend to be much happier with residents who have introduced themselves, examined patients in the preoperative holding room, and posted films in the operating room before they get there than one who arrives 5 minutes before the case is scheduled to start. Managing where you need to be can be difficult at times, as schedule changes and coverage issues often arise. Being proactive and anticipating potential problems will minimize your chances of appearing irresponsible to those expecting you.

RULE #4: BE PREPARED FOR ALL CONFERENCES AND YOUR OPERATIVE CASES

This will obviously improve what you get out of your day-to-day activities. You will definitely learn more sitting in a lecture or conference having read the assigned material than trying to passively absorb the discussion. Keep up with your academic schedule, reviewing the text and reading journal articles a few days in advance rather than trying to cram it in the night before. With respect to your operative cases, it is recommended that you have a plan written out for every case in which you assist. This should include the surgical approach and relevant anatomy, reduction technique, anticipated implants, and potential complications to look out for. Tape a copy of your written plan next to the x-rays if necessary. By being well prepared, you will undoubtedly get more out of the case. Also, more times than not, the attending will take notice and award you more responsibility during the procedure.

RULE #5: ALWAYS BE AVAILABLE

Keep your cell phone and beeper on at all times, both in and out of the hospital. This will let everyone you work with, both fellow residents and attendings, know that you can be depended on both day and night. Situations may arise when you have information vital to patient care that other members of your team need, and the ability to get in touch with you is important. On days when your schedule is light, try to avoid the urge to run out of the hospital. Being around, scrubbing on extra cases, or helping out in clinic can help your fellow residents get through a tough day while providing you with a worthwhile educational experience you would have otherwise missed out on.

RULE #6: IF THERE IS ANY UNCERTAINTY ABOUT YOUR PATIENT, CHECK X-RAYS AND LABS AND CALL THE ATTENDING OR CHIEF RESIDENT

The corollary to this rule is that you can *never* be certain. It is almost universally true that the more painful course of action for you will be the right one to do for your patients. Getting a page at 3:00 am from the nurse regarding inadequate pain control in your postoperative patient should not be managed with a reflexive response to increase the analgesic dose. Pulling yourself out of bed to examine the patient and confirm that the compartments are soft and that they are neurologically intact is a must. Whether it is 4:00 in the afternoon or 4:00 in the morning, when complicated situations arise that you are unsure about, the best practice is to pick up the phone and call your senior or the attending. No one will ever fault you for going the extra mile for a patient's well-being.

RULE #7: MAINTAIN PERSPECTIVE

Working in the hospital day in and day out can sometimes make it easy to lose sight of the fact that we are taking care of people who have entrusted us with their health, function, and well-being. Remember that whether it be a clinic visit or an operative procedure, it is likely an anxiety-provoking time for the patient and his or her family. Professionalism requires us to avoid rushing through a clinic visit or joking around with our fellow residents during rounds or in the operating room. Keeping a "big picture" attitude toward your training will improve your interaction with patients and the level of care you provide.

RULE #8: BE NICE AND RESPECTFUL TO THE ANCILLARY STAFF

Although this may seem like another common sense rule, it is one that needs to be emphasized. Only good things will come out of being polite and respectful to everyone you work with. This is true down the line from the nursing staff, operating room scrub technicians, x-ray techs, and the attending's office staff. Besides making the work environment much more pleasant, good relationships with the ancillary staff will likely lead them to go the extra mile for you if need be. You never know where you will be after you finish your residency training or whom you will be getting your patient referrals from. Being known as a nice person in addition to a talented physician will be more beneficial to you than being known as an obnoxious, short-tempered resident. Keep in mind the old saying, "you attract more bees with honey than you do with vinegar," and you will be happier with the results.

RULE #9: NEVER WHINE OR COMPLAIN TO SENIORS

Try to never forget that this was the path that you spent all of those long hours studying trying to get to. At times, being an orthopedic surgery resident can be a lot to handle and even draining—days when it seems you live at the hospital, where you spent countless hours covering 20 ER consults (8 of which are for pus) and 12 hours "holding the hooks" on a front-back spine case. Fight the urge to whine about it—especially to your senior residents. They were in your shoes and know what it is like to be a junior resident. Coming from two senior residents, trust us that others do not want to re-live the hardships through your complaining. Without a doubt, during your 4 years of training, you will need to vent from time to time. Do so with your classmates—those who are going through the same struggle. Together, you will get through the rough times and enjoy the better times.

RULE #10: READ AS MUCH AS HUMANLY POSSIBLE

There is a tremendous amount of material to learn during your training. Learning operative techniques through scrubbing cases is of utmost importance, but residency is more than a simple apprenticeship. The more you read, the better off you (and your future patients) will be. Try to make a reading schedule early in residency—starting out with textbooks and progressing on to review books and journal articles. Studying for the Orthopaedic In-Training Exam (OITE) and your board exam will be a much better experience (and less stressful) if you have developed a strong foundation and knowledge base early on. This point cannot be stressed enough—whenever possible, sit down and read. Read between cases. Sacrifice an hour of sleep on call to go over a single topic. Read for an hour each night before bed. Conditioning yourself to be a good student of orthopedic surgery will benefit you throughout your training and will continue once you are out in the real world.

RECOMMENDED TEXTS FOR YOUR PERSONAL LIBRARY

General Orthopedics

Canale ST, Beaty JH. *Campbell's Operative Orthopaedics*. 11th ed. Philadelphia, PA: Mosby Elsevier; 2008.

Fischgrund JS. *Orthopaedic Knowledge Update 9*. Rosemont, IL: American Academy of Orthopaedic Surgeons; 2008.

Hoppenfeld S, DeBoer P. *Surgical Exposures in Orthopaedics: The Anatomic Approach*. 3rd ed. Philadelphia, PA: Lippincott Williams & Wilkins; 2003.

Miller MD. *Review of Orthopaedics*. 5th ed. Philadelphia, PA: Saunders; 2008.

Spivak JM, Di Cesare PE, Feldman DS, Koval KJ, Rokito AS, Zuckerman JD. *Orthopaedics: A Study Guide*. New York, NY: McGraw-Hill; 1999.

Adult Reconstruction

Callaghan JJ, Rosenberg AG, Rubash HE. *The Adult Hip*. Philadelphia, PA: Lippincott Williams & Wilkins; 1998.

Scott WN. *Insall & Scott Surgery of the Knee*. 4th ed. New York, NY: Churchill Livingstone; 2006.

HAND/ELBOW

Green D, Hotchkiss R, Pederson WC. *Green's Operative Hand Surgery*. 5th ed. New York, NY: Churchill Livingstone; 2005.

Morrey BF. *Elbow and Its Disorders*. 3rd ed. Philadelphia, PA: WB Saunders; 2000.

PEDIATRIC ORTHOPEDICS

Morrissy RT, Weinstein SL. *Lovell and Winter's Pediatric Orthopaedics*. 6th ed. Philadelphia, PA: Lippincott Williams & Wilkins; 2006.

SHOULDER

Iannotti JP, Williams GR. *Disorders of the Shoulder: Diagnosis and Management*. Philadelphia, PA: Lippincott Williams & Wilkins; 1999.

SPORTS MEDICINE

DeLee JC, Drez D, Jr., Miller MD. *Delee and Drez's Orthopaedic Sports Medicine: Principles and Practice*. 2nd ed. Philadelphia, PA: WB Saunders; 2003.

Miller MD, Cole BD. *Textbook of Arthroscopy*. Philadelphia, PA: WB Saunders; 2004.

TRAUMA

Beaty JH, Kasser JR. *Rockwood and Wilkins' Fractures in Children*. 6th ed. Philadelphia, PA: Lippincott Williams & Wilkins; 2006.

Browner B, Levine A, Jupiter J, Trafton P, Krettek C. *Skeletal Trauma: Basic Science, Management, and Reconstruction*. 4th ed. Philadelphia, PA: Saunders; 2008.

Bucholz RW, Heckman JD, Court-Brown CM, Tornetta P, Koval KJ. *Rockwood and Green's Fractures in Adults*. 6th ed. Philadelphia, PA: Lippincott Williams & Wilkins; 2006.

Wiss DA. *Masters Techniques in Orthopaedic Surgery: Fractures*. 2nd ed. Philadelphia, PA: Lippincott Williams & Wilkins; 2006.

TUMOR

Wold LE, Adler CP, Sim FH, Unni KK. *Atlas of Orthopedic Pathology*. 2nd ed. Philadelphia, PA: WB Saunders; 2002.

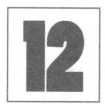

PROGRAM AND INSTITUTIONAL REQUIREMENTS

The Accreditation Council for Graduate Medical Education (ACGME) is the accrediting body for all residency programs for all specialties that are members of the American Board of Medical Specialties (ABMS). Each specialty has a Residency Review Committee (RRC) that is responsible for reviewing all residency programs within that specialty. The RRC for orthopedic surgery is responsible for monitoring each residency program through site visits that take place at least every 5 years and frequently at shorter intervals. Site visits are performed by experienced personnel who may or may not be orthopedic surgeons. However, all members of the orthopedic surgery RRC are orthopedic surgeons.

There are two types of "requirements" specified by the ACGME. The first represents institutional requirements, and these specify the resources and policies and procedures that each institution must provide if they are to be accredited to sponsor residency training of any type. These are referred to as *institutional requirements*. For example, the New York University School of Medicine is the sponsoring institution for the NYU Hospital for Joint Diseases Orthopaedic Surgery Residency Program. Therefore, the NYU School of Medicine also undergoes periodic site visits to confirm that it provides the institutional resources and has the policies and procedures in place to support the numerous residency programs it sponsors.

In addition, each residency program must fulfill the *program requirements* specific for that area of training. Program requirements will differ for each residency program depending on the specialty. However, institutional requirements are the same for any institution that sponsors residency programs regardless of the number or types of programs and the institution's location and size. Detailed descriptions of institutional and program requirements are available on the ACGME Web site at www.acgme.org. Although most of this chapter will focus primarily on the program requirements for orthopedic surgery, I will start with a description of some of the relevant institutional responsibilities.

Joseph D. Zuckerman, MD

L. M. Jazrawi, K. A. Egol, & J. D. Zuckerman.
Orthopedic Residency & Fellowship: A Guide to Success (pp. 75-78)
© 2010 Taylor & Francis Group.

An important emphasis of the institutional requirements is on the institution's commitment to graduate medical education. The requirements specify that the "sponsored institution must insure that program directors have sufficient financial support and protected time to effectively carry out their educational and administrative responsibilities to their respective programs."[1] This is important because it emphasizes that each residency program director must have the support necessary to direct the program. The institutional requirements also indicate that the sponsoring institution "must assure that residents are provided with a written letter of appointment/contract outlining the terms and conditions of their appointment to the program"[1] and that when problems arise, the sponsoring institution must "provide residents with fair, reasonable, and readily available written institutional policies and procedures for grievance and due process."[1] The institutional requirements also address issues related to moonlighting, counseling services, physician impairment, harassment, and accommodation of disabilities. They also emphasize that each sponsoring institution "must ensure a healthy and safe work environment that provides for food services, call rooms and adequate security and safety."[1] As noted, the details of the ACGME institutional requirements can be reviewed at www.acgme.org.

Fulfilling the ACGME Program Requirements for Graduate Medical Education in Orthopaedic Surgery is essential for a residency program to maintain accreditation. The program requirements include specific requirements for orthopedic surgery as well as a set of common program requirements that apply to each residency program. The actual program requirements are 22 pages in length and are updated periodically to reflect changes in orthopedic residency education.[2] The most recent update as of this writing was July 1, 2007. In this section, we will highlight some of these requirements.

The ACGME defines orthopedic surgery as the "medical specialty that includes the study and prevention of musculoskeletal diseases, disorders and injuries and their treatment by medical, surgical and physical methods."[2] A 5-year residency program is required with specific rotations required for the first post-graduate year (PGY-1) year. The PGY-1 year must include a minimum of 6 months of structured education in surgery to include multisystem trauma, plastic surgery/burn care, intensive care, and vascular surgery; a minimum of 1 month of structured education in at least 3 of the following: emergency medicine, medical/cardiac intensive care, internal medicine, neurology/neurological surgery, pediatric surgery or pediatrics, rheumatology, anesthesiology, musculoskeletal imaging, and rehabilitation; and a maximum of 3 months of orthopedic surgery.

The residency program director is also responsible for the design, implementation, and oversight of the PGY-2 through PGY-5 years that "must include at least three years of rotations in orthopedic services and may include rotations on related services, such as plastic surgery, physical medicine and rehabilitation, rheumatology, or neurological surgery."[2] In practice, almost every program includes orthopedic rotations throughout the PGY-2 through PGY-5 years, although many programs include elective and research rotations.

The RRC allows multiple sites for training as long as one site provides most of the residents' basic science and research education, as well as providing extensive clinical experience. Other sites of training must fulfill specific requirements related to the number of teaching faculty, duration and content of the educational experience, and the level of supervision in the program. In addition, each residency program must have a single program director. The ACGME goes on to specify the qualifications and the responsibilities of the Residency Program Director. This is a very important area to which the ACGME devotes 4 pages of their program requirements to define the responsibilities of the program director related to resident education, supervision, evaluations, work hours, documentation, and research. Included in this is the responsibility of the program director to "ensure that faculty and residents attend and participate in regularly scheduled teaching rounds, lectures and conferences."[2] In addition to the program director, each program is required to have a sufficient number of teaching faculty "to instruct and supervise all residents at a specific location."[2] Specifically, there must be at least one full-time faculty equivalent (1 FTE=45 hours per week devoted to the residency) for every 4 residents in the program. And all programs must have at least 3 faculty members who contribute at least 20 hours per week to the residency program. The faculty involved in the program "must establish and maintain an environment of inquiry and scholarship with an active research component."[2] The program requirements go on to specify that some members of the faculty should also demonstrate scholarship as evidenced by peer-reviewed funding, publication of original research, publication and presentations at local, regional, and national meetings, and participation in national committees or educational organizations.

As expected, the program requirements contain an extensive description of the educational program that should be provided in each residency program. These include the overall educational goals and objectives for the program, which should be distributed annually to all residents and faculty. Competency-based goals and objectives for each resident rotation at each educational level must also be distributed annually to residents and faculty. The ACGME competencies are emphasized and defined in detail, including patient care, medical knowledge, practice-based learning and improvement, interpersonal communication skills, professionalism, and systems-based practice. The 6 competencies have become the foundation of resident education in this country and is the common thread among all residency training programs.

The evaluation of the residents and the program are also important components of residency training. The faculty are required to "evaluate resident performance in a timely manner during each rotation and these evaluations must be accessible for review by each resident."[2] Similarly, the faculty of each program must be evaluated annually, not only by the program director, but also by the residents. The confidential nature of these evaluations is stressed. Residents should also evaluate the residency program with respect to the education and experience provided, and the program is required to use these evaluations to improve the program.

The ACGME also specifies the minimal passing rate for the Part I and Part II American Board of Orthopaedic Surgery (ABOS) exams. The requirements indicate that "program graduates should take both Part I and Part II of the ABOS exams and at least 75% of those who take the exams for the first time should pass."[2]

As expected, the program requirements also provide extensive documentation of the resident duty hour requirements, supervision, fatigue issues, and moonlighting. These are requirements that are common to all residency programs regardless of specialty.

Residency training in orthopedic surgery is a 5-year experience in which each resident should develop the knowledge and experience to successfully complete the ABOS exams and to enter the practice of orthopedic surgery. Monitoring of the orthopedic residency programs by the ACGME is an essential part of accreditation, and each residency program works diligently to fulfill the program requirements. As you evaluate residency programs, the results of previous RRC site visits can be informative with respect to the quality of the education provided and the responsiveness of the program in addressing any potential areas of deficiency.

REFERENCES

1. Accreditation Council for Graduate Medical Education. ACGME institutional requirements. 2007. Available at: http://www.acgme.org/acWebsite/irc/irc_IRCpr07012007.pdf. Accessed December 15, 2009.
2. Accreditation Council for Graduate Medical Education. ACGME program requirements for graduate medical education in orthopaedic surgery. 2007. Available at: http://www.acgme.org/acWebsite/downloads/RRC_progReq/260orthopaedicsurgery07012007.pdf. Accessed December 15, 2009.

WOMEN IN ORTHOPEDIC SURGERY

While women comprise approximately 50% of each medical school class, the number applying to the field of orthopedic surgery is significantly less. In fact, the percentage of women in orthopedics remained constant between 1998 and 2001.[1] The most recent statistic according to the Fellowship and Residency Electronic Interactive Database (FREIDA) Web site notes that the current percentage of female orthopedic surgery residents and fellows is 11.4%. It is not known whether to attribute this discrepancy to lack of interest, lack of proper mentoring, or other factors; however, it is a very real phenomenon. Most women considering the field of orthopedics as a career have spent time immersed in the culture and generally understand, accept, and even value their minority status. There are, however, certain aspects of this role that are difficult to recognize prior to entering the field. This guide will hopefully elucidate some of these factors. Regardless of gender, orthopedic surgery attracts the best and the brightest medical students, and it takes drive, determination, educational excellence, and research interest to be considered for an interview.

STARTING FROM THE BEGINNING

MENTORSHIP

As a female medical student interested in orthopedics, it is helpful to seek out female mentors in the field to facilitate increased exposure to the specialty. Valuable foresight into subjects such as residency and fellowship training, surgical cases, lifestyle, private practice versus academics, and family life may be addressed with your mentor. Mentors need not be attending orthopedic surgeons. Valuable information may be gathered from female residents and fellows currently going through the process. There are many career and lifestyle issues that are easier to discuss with other women.

Suezie Kim, MD and Catherine Laible, MD

L. M. Jazrawi, K. A. Egol, & J. D. Zuckerman.
Orthopedic Residency & Fellowship: A Guide to Success (pp. 79-82)
© 2010 Taylor & Francis Group.

EXCEL

As a woman in a predominantly male field, you will always stand out. The key is to embrace this and use it to your benefit to make your mark and excel. It is undoubtedly acceptable not to be "one of the guys." It is also certainly a positive to have multiple women in a program and be able to be "one of the girls." Regardless, academic excellence is always the key to success in competitive residency programs. Medicine has always been a "meritocracy" and as such, candidates with an outstanding academic, research, and community service background will always stand out.

NOW THAT YOU'VE MADE THE DECISION TO APPLY TO ORTHOPEDICS

Despite the inherent differences between men and women, the application process in orthopedic surgery is the same. Of course, you should work for the highest grades possible, striving particularly for honors in your clinical and orthopedic elective clerkships. Quality letters of recommendation are essential, and great mentors can lead to very personal, strong letters. Research experience is commonly looked upon as a necessity in the field of orthopedics, and in-depth projects and publications can often make the difference between two well-qualified candidates. Away rotations are essential, and how you perform during these can often make or break your interview invitation to a particular program.

STRENGTH IN NUMBERS

For any woman applying in orthopedics, you reach an understanding within yourself that the possibility exists of being the only woman or one of a few women in a program. While you may get along with and share similar interests with your male co-residents, having other women around who are going through a similar experience is invaluable. A program with multiple women is also more likely to be open to accepting more women.

YOU MADE IT!

Postgraduate medical education invokes many emotions regardless of the specialty chosen. Whether it is excitement, joy, disbelief, anticipation, or trepidation, residency is the next stage in a journey of lifelong education. You are now able to practice medicine and begin the path to becoming an orthopedic surgeon. As a female resident in orthopedics, there are certain hurdles to be conscious of that many of your male colleagues may be unaware of.

PERCEPTIONS

The specialty of orthopedic surgery invokes many stereotypes, both positive and negative. Women in orthopedics are certainly not excluded from this. Not all women in orthopedic surgery are tall, muscular, former athletes. Many orthopedic residency programs across the country by now have accepted women; however, it is important to remember that every person you meet while applying, interviewing, and during your training and practice will have a different perception of you. Starting with your decision to apply to orthopedics and continuing throughout your career, keep in mind that you can either change or support these perceptions, and your actions affect how people you meet view women in general within the field.

BE YOURSELF, BE PROFESSIONAL

In a program surrounded with men, it is understandable to feel uncomfortable acting like a woman. Residency is demanding and challenging enough. Embrace who you are, not who you think you should be. While most of your colleagues may not understand the stress relief in a post-call manicure or therapeutic hair appointment, feeling like the woman you are is essential to your well-being.

INTERNSHIP

A general surgical internship is currently required for those entering orthopedic surgery. Most programs now incorporate at least 3 months of orthopedic rotations in addition to the various general surgery requirements as well as rotations in other subspecialties such as radiology, anesthesia, intensive care, emergency medicine, and rheumatology. Women are commonly found in many of these associated specialties; use this as a chance to make great friendships that you'll be able to rely on for the many years ahead of you. This is also a good time to review the basics of orthopedics, including anatomy and general pathology. A broad basis of knowledge gathered during internship will prove indispensable for your residency. This year also provides a great opportunity to explore the city that you live in, find a nearby gym, make new friends, and eat some good food.

RESIDENCY

The second post-graduate year (PGY-2; first-year orthopedics) is the beginning of your chosen career path. Your rotations are now with your fellow orthopedic residents and with your department faculty and staff. You will now treat orthopedic patients, perform their surgeries, and learn about their pathologies. It is an exciting time with a great deal of new information and constant learning. All programs have didactic lectures and labs built into the curriculum; however, you must also learn independently as well. Residency is a great opportunity to make your mark within your chosen specialty. You will begin to build a reputation for yourself as well as start to network within the orthopedic community. Relationships made here will likely last you throughout your career. Mentorship continues through residency. It is important to find a strong mentor within your department or through your institution's graduate medical education council.

PUTTING IT ALL TOGETHER

As a woman in a field dominated by men, you will find that you are treated differently. It may be as obvious as patients mistaking you for the nurse, or as subtle as not finishing up a conversation with your male colleague because you have to change in a different locker room. Although you may encounter some frustrating situations, it is vital that you turn those into an opportunity to shine. Always remember to be professional and courteous, and address the issue at hand in a composed manner. Look forward to the times when a female orthopedist is sought out by patients. There are many patients, particularly women, who appreciate being seen, examined, and operated on by us.

Residency is not all about work. Many residents, both men and women, find time to be with family and friends, meet new people, enjoy recreational sports, and even have children. It is imperative to stay grounded and enjoy life outside of medicine. Taking care of your own mind and body allows you to be the best physician for your patients.

The road to residency and the journey through it is just a small part of your career as a woman in orthopedic surgery. There are innumerable facets of medicine and life; it is inevitable that you will encounter great joys as well as difficulties. Work hard, don't complain, be proactive, and be yourself. Remember that many women have gone through this journey prior to you, and it is often helpful to find someone to talk to.

REFERENCE

1. Templeton K, Wood VJ, Haynes R. Women and minorities in orthopedic residency programs. *JAAOS*. 2007;15(suppl 1):S37-S41.

RECOMMENDED READING

American Medical Association. FRIEDA online. Available at: http://www.ama-assn.org/ama/pub/education-careers/graduate-medical-education/freida-online.shtml. Accessed November 18, 2009.

Biermann JS. Women in orthopedic surgery residencies in the United States. *Academic Medicine.* 1998;73(6):708-709.

Blakemore LC, Hall JM, Biermann JS. Women in surgical residency training programs. *J Bone Joint Surg Am.* 2003;85A(12):2477-2480.

Gebhardt MC. Improving diversity in orthopaedic residency programs. *JAAOS.* 2007; 15(suppl 1):S49-S50.

Ruth Jackson Orthopaedic Society. Web site. Available at: http://www.rjos.org/web/index.html. Accessed November 18, 2009.

Scherl SA, Lively N, Simon MA. Initial review of Electronic Residency Application Service charts by orthopaedic residency faculty members. Does applicant gender matter? *J Bone Joint Surg Am.* 2001;83A(1):65-70.

THE ORTHOPAEDIC IN-TRAINING EXAM

The Orthopaedic In-Training Exam (OITE) is distributed by the American Academy of Orthopaedic Surgeons (AAOS) on an annual basis to all residents training in programs accredited by the Accreditation Council for Graduate Medical Education (ACGME). The first ever OITE exam, consisting of 150 multiple-choice questions, was administered to 1,118 residents in 171 programs in November 1963.[1] The current OITE has evolved since then and now consists of 275 multiple-choice questions designed to cover 12 defined content domains spanning musculoskeletal basic sciences and all of the subspecialties of orthopedic surgery.

This mandatory annual examination is designed to serve as an educational aid and impetus for residents to continuously study musculoskeletal basic sciences and clinical orthopedics during each year of residency. Results should provide residents with a means of tracking the growth of their fund of knowledge on an annual basis and the ability to compare their performances with peers across the country in the same year of postgraduate training. Furthermore, the annual results provide residency program directors and active faculty members standardized data about the performance of their program—overall and by year of training—relative to other ACGME-accredited training programs. Therefore, results should be used by the individual resident to adjust self-learning behaviors and by programs to refine and continually improve their didactic programs.

The OITE will also serve as an early assessment of your preparedness for the American Board of Orthopaedic Surgery (ABOS) Part 1 written examination, which is taken in July following residency graduation. Studies have shown OITE scores to be predictive of ABOS Part I performance. For example, a 2004 review of all graduates from a single institution over 10 years showed that all residents who failed the ABOS Part 1 scored lower than the 30th percentile on the OITE during the third and fourth post-graduate years (PGY-3 and PGY-4), and below the 27th percentile during their final year.[2] In a more recent study, another institution analyzed graduates over a 10-year period and found that those who failed the ABOS Part 1 received a mean percentile score of 32 on the OITE during their PGY-2, PGY-3, and PGY-4 years and a mean percentile of 30 on their PGY-5 OITE.[3]

Eric J. Strauss, MD and David E. Ruchelsman, MD

L. M. Jazrawi, K. A. Egol, & J. D. Zuckerman.
Orthopedic Residency & Fellowship: A Guide to Success (pp. 83-86)
© 2010 Taylor & Francis Group.

Chapter 14

EXAM PREPARATION

We emphasize that the preparation for the OITE examination, ABOS Part 1 written examination, and a successful career in orthopedic surgery really begins on the first day of the orthopedic internship. As a result of this, our department has recently instituted an orthopedic core curriculum for our PGY-1 residents. A weekly didactic session is mandated for all of our interns to introduce them to the fundamental principles of the specialty throughout the first 12 months of training. This time is considered protected "required education" time—that is, our interns are excused from their clinical duties to attend these important sessions. We believe this will serve as an essential bridge to the formal start of the orthopedic training program in the PGY-2 year.

All accredited orthopedic residency programs are required by the Residency Review Committee (RRC) and ACGME to provide clinical and basic science education each academic year in anticipation of the annual OITE. We stress that the dedicated OITE review sessions are by no means a substitute for the self-directed study that each resident is expected to complete. Mandatory core readings on each subspecialty rotation, specialty-based weekly conferences, and nightly preparation for operative cases serve as the building blocks for academic success.

As time is often limited by clinical responsibilities, a structured study schedule made several months in advance of the OITE that allows for frequent review of the material is essential. Study materials should include core readings from previous subspecialty rotations (textbook chapters and journal articles), notes from service-based conferences, and various review materials. Reviewing questions from prior examinations becomes helpful once one has reviewed all of the content. Materials that residents in our program have found helpful in preparation for the OITE include the following:

- ✓ *Miller's Review of Orthopaedics*, 5th ed, Saunders/Elsevier, Philadelphia, 2008: This is an excellent review text; however, it can be overwhelming for junior residents as it presumes a fundamental knowledge base. It is mostly used by senior residents.

- ✓ *Orthopaedics: A Study Guide*, McGraw-Hill, New York, 1999 and *Orthopaedic Knowledge Update* (OKU) published by AAOS: These are individual subspecialty review books that are excellent sources of information and can be used on each subspecialty rotation.

- ✓ *Review articles*: Review articles can be found in various journals. These include the *Journal of the American Academy of Orthopaedic Surgeons* (JAAOS), Instructional Course Lectures (ICLs) and Current Concepts articles published in the *Journal of Bone and Joint Surgery* (JBJS), *Clinical Orthopaedics and Related Research*, *Journal of Hand Surgery* (JHS), *Journal of Shoulder and Elbow Surgery* (JSES), and *American Journal of Sports Medicine* (AJSM), to name a few. These reviews are read throughout the year to build knowledge as one sees consults and outpatients, and in preparation for operative cases.

- ✓ *Orthopaedic Self-Interest Examinations (OSIEs)/Self-Assessment Examinations*: Published by AAOS, 6300 North River Road, Rosemont, IL 60018; (847)-823-7186; www4.aaos.org/product/products.cfm. The OSIEs are distributed by the AAOS annually. Each annual edition covers 3 separate specialties and is an excellent resource. The 9 subspecialties are therefore covered over a 3-year cycle. These are challenging and are designed for those preparing for maintenance of certification and those in practice seeking CME credit.

✓ *Previous OITEs*: Reviewing prior examinations is helpful to begin to understand content covered and the types of questions to anticipate on the examination. Several questions, or variations on them, tend to repeat each year. Recognizing and understanding wrong answers on previous tests will help you answer new questions correctly. Our residents compile detailed explanations for each question and highlight the core content related to each answer choice; this provides a detailed syllabus for thorough review of a significant amount of information with each examination reviewed. Further, using our new Web-based educational model, Advanced Learning Exchange (ALEX), questions in each prior examination are now divided by topic (ie, anatomy, trauma, pediatric orthopedics, orthopedic pathology, etc), which affords each resident the opportunity to individualize his or her study programs using this extensive bank of questions.

WEB SITES

Journal of Bone and Joint Surgery: www.ejbjs.org
Journal of the American Academy of Orthopaedic Surgeons: www.jaaos.org
Orthopedics Hyperguide: www.ortho.hyperguides.com
Orthopaedic Knowledge Online: www5.aaos.org/oko/login.cfm

TEST-TAKING STRATEGIES

1. If you don't know an answer, guess—always. (You are not penalized for wrong answers.)
2. Beware of answers with absolutes such as "always" or "100% of cases."
3. Use information obtained from other questions and photographs on the exam.
4. Be logical.
5. Train yourself to guess the answer before you look at the choices.
6. If the correct answer is not immediately apparent, begin by eliminating answers that are obviously wrong.
7. Don't waste time on any question whose answer completely eludes you; a quick guess is better.
8. Keep in mind that all questions have the same point value.
9. Suppress the urge to change an answer in response to an afterthought—it is usually less accurate than your first thought.
10. Consider only the information given; don't "read into" the question.

In conclusion, study regularly, identify your strengths and weaknesses by taking previous OITEs, and read the resources listed above throughout your residency.

REFERENCES

1. Nattress LW, Jr. Orthopaedic In-Training Examination. *J Med Educ*. 1969;44:878.
2. Klein GR, Austin MS, Randolph S, Sharkey PF, Hilibrand AS. Passing the boards: can USMLE and Orthopaedic In-Training Examination scores predict passage of the ABOS Part-I examination? *J Bone Joint Surg Am*. 2004;86:1092-1095.
3. Herndon JH, Allan BJ, Dyer G, Jawa A, Zurakowski D. Predictors of success on the American Board of Orthopaedic Surgery Examination. *Clin Orthop Relat Res*. E-pub ahead of print, June 26, 2009.

RESEARCH DURING YOUR RESIDENCY

The importance of evidence-based practice is increasing within orthopedic surgery. The Accreditation Council for Graduate Medical Education (ACGME) requires orthopedic residents to participate in scholarly activity, and as such, most orthopedic residency programs require their residents to take part in research activities. Regardless of requirements, programs believe that participation in clinical and basic science research as a resident will develop the skills necessary to contribute to and critically evaluate advances within the field. In addition to the long hours spent providing patient care, taking call, and preparing for your operative cases, completing a research project that leads to publication in a peer-reviewed journal can be a difficult but rewarding endeavor. By adding to the literature, your efforts will potentially provide clinicians with new information or techniques that can impact outcomes for orthopedic surgery patients. Additionally, success on the academic side of orthopedics through research will strengthen your ability to secure the fellowship or job of your choice. The considerable time and effort necessary to take a research project from an idea to publication requires one to get started early on in training.

GETTING STARTED

Two of the most important aspects of getting your research efforts going are picking a topic worth investigating and finding a faculty member to act as your research mentor. It is often a good idea to choose a research issue within the subspecialty you think you will pursue, as this will keep you motivated and interested while being beneficial on your application for fellowship. Your involvement in a particular clinical scenario might trigger an idea for a research study, or a review of recently published articles may allow you to formulate a research question that has not been adequately answered. Additionally, academically productive faculty members at your institution typically have multiple ongoing studies and research ideas that you can get involved in if you ask. Last, in reviewing the topic and research question, you will become a relative expert in the field in terms of the knowledge and background of the material. This will undoubtedly assist in your mastery of the clinical condition as well.

Eric J. Strauss, MD and David E. Ruchelsman, MD

L. M. Jazrawi, K. A. Egol, & J. D. Zuckerman.
Orthopedic Residency & Fellowship: A Guide to Success (pp. 87-92)
© 2010 Taylor & Francis Group.

It is never too early in your residency training to get the wheels moving with regard to research. During your first post-graduate year (PGY-1) or PGY-2, find a faculty member within your department with whom you feel that you can work well and express interest in getting started in a study. Choose your mentor carefully, as working with an attending who has a good track record of getting studies finished and published is much more rewarding than working with a faculty member who is slow to review your work and contribute. Scrambling as a PGY-4 to begin a research effort in order to bolster your fellowship application or as a chief resident trying to quickly complete your research requirement will be unpleasant and unlikely to produce a quality result. Whether you decide to engage in an ongoing study your faculty mentor has started or come up with a novel idea or clinical problem to investigate, picking your topic is the important first step.

Next, set up a reasonable timeline for each step of your study with the goal of getting your hard work published in a quality orthopedic surgery journal. Retrospective clinical studies can often be accomplished quickly while collecting data in a prospective clinical investigation may take considerably longer. If you choose a basic science or biomechanical study, it is a good idea to get a feel for the time that will be required to obtain the specimens you need and perform the testing as this will obviously impact your ability to complete your study in a timely fashion. Review your planned timeline with your faculty mentor and get started as soon as possible.

THE LITERATURE REVIEW

Once you have chosen an idea or a particular research question to be investigated, your next step is to perform a thorough literature search. This will enable you to determine what work has been previously done on your topic and significantly increase your knowledge base. It also allows you to confirm that your study hasn't already been performed elsewhere.

Using PubMed (www.ncbi.nlm.nih.gov/pubmed), you can identify related studies on your topic through various combinations of keyword searches. Closely examine these related studies for their materials and methods, which will enable you to determine what is "standard" for your type of research project. Although variability will undoubtedly exist in each published study, knowledge of the patient demographic information collected, radiographic evaluations used, surgical approaches included, and specific outcome scoring systems used in the postoperative assessment will help you in the structuring of your investigation and paper. Once you have read these related papers, you will be able to confirm the feasibility of your planned research project and understand the type of information and analysis required for acceptance into a peer-reviewed orthopedic journal.

Subsequent to your literature review, it is a good idea to start writing an outline for your manuscript (covered in greater detail below). Based on the information that you've gathered from reading the related papers, the introduction and materials and methods sections may be started. While these sections will likely change and evolve as your project continues, getting the manuscript started will allow you to clearly and concisely define the goals of the project and will save you time later in the process.

INSTITUTIONAL REVIEW BOARD APPROVAL

Every research project needs to be approved by your hospital's Institutional Review Board (IRB), which can be a lengthy and time-consuming process in its own right.

Although this may seem unnecessary for certain types of studies such as chart reviews and retrospective investigations, many journals now require that every manuscript include a statement that the reported research received IRB approval.

The IRB application and requirements vary at each institution but typically require a description of your study goals, the involved investigators, inclusion and exclusion criteria, proposed methods, samples of informed consent forms, and proof of a proper literature search. Because you have already completed your literature search and written the introduction and materials and methods section of your manuscript, completing the IRB application should not be a problem.

POWER ANALYSIS

Likely, the IRB application will require inclusion of a power analysis for your study and the involvement of a statistician early is often necessary. A power analysis is a statistical procedure for determining the number of subjects that you need to enroll in your study to be able to detect a significant difference between the study variables. Details on performing a power analysis can be found in Kevin Freedman and Joseph Bernstein's article.[1]

If your institution has an in-house epidemiologist or statistician, it is a good idea for you to consult him or her for this portion of your study planning. He or she will be able to look at a few of the related studies that you found during your literature search or at data from a small pilot study and let you know how many subjects you need for your study to be successful. In addition to performing the power analysis, the epidemiologist can provide an important evaluation of your study design and will likely be more willing to help out in the data analysis later on in the process. This step is critical because if your study is underpowered or improperly designed, months of hard work may be wasted that could have been addressed at the very beginning.

DATA COLLECTION, SPECIMEN TESTING, AND ANALYSIS

Your study is nothing without data, and the process of collecting data or testing your specimens can be time consuming and painful if you are not organized and prepared. For clinical studies, you will likely be reviewing patient charts, office notes, and operative reports or conducting interviews and physical exams. Having a pre-prepared data collection sheet will allow you to be efficient while gathering all of the important information. Additionally, setting up a detailed Excel spreadsheet will help keep you organized and make data analysis easier once the data collection period is complete. For basic science and biomechanical studies, it is a good idea to get a feel for how long the set up and testing will take. This will allow you to dedicate enough time in your day to obtain the data you are looking for without wasting thawed specimens or valuable time on the testing machines.

Proper data analysis is critical to report the findings from your study, and unless you have a statistics background, it is a good idea to consult your hospital's epidemiologist or statistician for help. Depending on your study design, a number of different statistical tests can be used, and getting your paper by a journal's reviewers relies on choosing the correct ones.

PREPARING THE MANUSCRIPT

With all of the data collected and analyzed, it is time to put together the paper for publication where you will convey the findings of your research project to the orthopedic readership. As you have already written a significant portion of the introduction and materials and methods before you started collecting data, the rest of the manuscript should not be too difficult to complete. Under the guidance of your faculty research mentor, decide which journal your paper will be submitted to as this will impact the structure of the manuscript. Many journals have "Information for Authors" sections on their Web sites, which outline their preferred style, formatting, and method for referencing. Another possibility is to look at an issue of the journal and review a few articles to obtain this information.

Writing a scientific article has its own rules and technique. Under the "Recommended Reading" at the end of this chapter, a few good resources are listed to assist you in composing your paper. Additionally, courses are regularly presented at the annual meeting of the American Academy of Orthopaedic Surgeons (AAOS), providing insight into how a good research paper is written and how the review process works. A typical research paper will include an introduction, where the nature of the question or problem is outlined with a concise review of background information provided, followed by a statement of the goals of the study with an associated hypothesis. Next, the materials and methods section highlights the structure of the investigation, including patient demographics, inclusion and exclusion criteria, surgical procedural information or details about the specimen testing protocol, outcome assessment tools used, and methods for statistical analysis of the data. The results section reports the findings of the study, including statistical comparisons between treatment or specimen groups. Finally, the discussion section allows for the findings of your study to be compared to those reported in other papers within the literature. A common method for discussion is to answer 4 main questions: What have you found? What has been reported in other studies? How do these findings compare? What were the limitations to your study?

Most orthopedic surgery journals employ an online submission process. Once your paper is complete and ready for submission, carefully follow the instructions on the journal's Web site to ensure a smooth submission. Make sure that you take the time to review your paper, looking for details such as spelling errors, improper referencing, and issues with the manuscript's structure. A poorly presented paper, regardless of content, will be viewed negatively by the journal's reviewers. Upon receipt of your paper, the journal will send it to 2 or 3 consultant reviewers who will decide whether they consider it worthy of publication—a process that typically takes 2 to 3 months. Decisions from the journal include acceptance (usually with minor revisions necessary), provisional acceptance following major revisions, or rejection. Keep faculty mentors involved throughout all steps as they are ultimately responsible for the content of the manuscript.

After you hear back from the journal regarding your paper, most of the time you still have work to do. A common saying in research is that the last 10% of the work takes 90% of the time. Assuming that your manuscript is accepted on the condition of major or minor revisions, you will receive a numbered list of questions or issues from each reviewer. Your next task is to address these comments and make the necessary changes to the paper. When you are ready to resubmit your revised work, you are expected to respond in writing to each of the reviewer's points, indicating your thoughts on the comment and the resultant change to the text of the manuscript. It is obviously in your best interest to do this in a gracious and humble manner. The comments and suggestions made by the reviewers will often improve the quality of your paper, so keep an open mind during this process. It is not uncommon for a paper to go through this process multiple times prior to being published, so don't get frustrated because your goal has almost been reached.

OTHER BENEFITS

Besides getting your research published in a peer-reviewed orthopedic journal, you may also decide to submit the abstract from your paper for presentation at a national or regional meeting. The annual meetings of the American Academy of Orthopaedic Surgeons (AAOS), the American Orthopaedic Society for Sports Medicine (AOSSM), the Orthopaedic Trauma Association (OTA), the American Society for Surgery of the Hand (ASSH), and the Pediatric Orthopaedic Society of North America (POSNA) are great places for residents to present their research activity on a national level. Most residency programs encourage research endeavors by giving you time off and paying your way to present at these national meetings. Check each society's Web site for abstract submission deadlines and other details.

In conclusion, you should be familiar with your program's research requirements, and you should get involved with research as early as possible. Choose topics that interest you, and use this time to work closely with faculty members. Your efforts will give you the opportunity to make a meaningful contribution to orthopedic literature, and the experience itself will provide you with skills that can be invaluable to your future as an orthopedic surgeon.

REFERENCE

1. Freedman KB, Bernstein J. Current concepts review: Sample size and statistical power in clinical orthopaedic research. *J Bone Joint Surg Am.* 1999;81A:1454-1460.

RECOMMENDED READING

Cowell HR. Preparing manuscripts for publication in the *Journal of Bone and Joint Surgery*: responsibilities of authors and editors: a view from the editor of the American volume. *J Bone Joint Surg Am.* 1993;75A:456-463.

Gillespie LD, Gillespie WJ. Finding current evidence: search strategies and common databases. *CORR.* 2003;413:133-145.

Schunemann HJ, Bone L. Evidence-based orthopaedics: a primer. *CORR.* 2003;413:117-132.

Wright RW, Brand RA, Dunn W, Spindler KP. How to write a systematic review. *CORR.* 2007;455:23-29.

Wright TM, Buckwalter JA, Hayes WC. Writing for the *Journal of Orthopaedic Research. J Orthop Res.* 1999;17:459-466.

16

FINANCES DURING YOUR RESIDENCY

This chapter will only focus on issues that should be addressed during your training, which include the following:

✓ *Establishing an emergency fund*: You should have 3 to 6 months of your expenses in accounts such as a savings account, checking account, or money market account that can be easily accessed without penalty.

✓ *Paying down credit card debt*: Generally, it makes more sense to pay off high-interest rate debts (such as credit cards) than putting money into riskier investments.

✓ *Purchasing disability and life insurance*: This is a first line of defense against financial loss. Having the correct type and amount of insurance will allow you and your family to remain in your "own world." Therefore, before investing, you should purchase an "Own-Occupation" disability insurance policy, as well as a term life insurance policy with at least a $1,000,000 death benefit.

✓ *Investing in IRAs and/or other employer-sponsored plans.*

Of course, as you advance in your career, any insurance and investment products purchased during training should become part of an overall comprehensive financial plan.

PAYING OFF YOUR HIGH-INTEREST DEBTS

CREDIT CARDS

One way to meet expenses while establishing yourself is to use credit cards to pay for things that you want or need but cannot currently afford. Although this may be a reasonable way to finance your vacation or pay for unexpected expenses, it can often lead to overuse. In fact, as an orthopedic surgeon, you may receive numerous solicitations promoting credit cards with low introductory interest rates, generous spending limits, and cash-advance privileges that can be attained just by signing your name.

Lawrence B. Keller, CFP®, CLU, ChFC, RHU, LUTCF

L. M. Jazrawi, K. A. Egol, & J. D. Zuckerman.
Orthopedic Residency & Fellowship: A Guide to Success (pp. 93-110)
© 2010 Taylor & Francis Group.

It is best to pay your credit card balances in full each month to avoid paying any interest charges. However, if you must carry a balance, make sure your card has the lowest interest rate possible or apply for a low-rate credit card that allows you to transfer your current balance to it.

Unfortunately, banks and other credit card companies don't have any real incentive to automatically lower your rate. However, if you have made your payments on time and call to ask for a lower rate, you will often be rewarded. This can save you hundreds to thousands of dollars over time.

However, be aware that having too many credit cards open could reduce your ability to qualify for a mortgage or other loan. Banks view your available credit as outstanding debt, even if you never charge what you could. Therefore, if you qualify for $100,000 in credit and have the ability to charge up to $15,000 already, you might only qualify for an additional $85,000. The more credit you have access to, the larger the problem you might have in the future. For this reason, you should remember to cancel the card if you don't plan on using it after you make the balance transfer.

If you find that credit cards are too dangerous for you due to a lack of self-discipline, try a debit card that draws directly on your bank account. Although you do not benefit by having the short-term loan features of a credit card, the convenience is retained (Table 16-1).

Other important things to consider:

✓ Understand the terms under which a card is issued.

✓ Sign all cards as soon as they are received.

✓ Keep detailed records of credit card account numbers, expiration dates, and the telephone number of the card issuer. The easiest way to do this is to make a photocopy of the front and back of each card.

✓ Carefully review your statement each month for accuracy.

PURCHASE DISABILITY AND LIFE INSURANCE COVERAGE

Purchasing adequate insurance protection is a fundamental component of a physician's financial plan. The purpose of insurance is to protect against risks that would be financially devastating to you and/or your family. Here, the risks of many individuals are transferred to an insurance company or other large group in return for a premium.

When it comes to insurance, unfortunately, most orthopedic surgeons don't pay much attention to details. They are more concerned about saving money in income taxes, investing in the stock market, or looking for new opportunities to increase their income beyond the practice of medicine. Unfortunately, this is equivalent to putting the roof on a house before its foundation has been laid.

During the past 20 years, the policies made available to orthopedic surgeons have continually changed. However, one thing has remained constant: Orthopedic surgeons at all stages of their careers, often unknowingly, make poor choices when it comes to protecting their most valuable asset—their ability to earn an income.

Table 16-1

ADVANTAGES AND DISADVANTAGES OF CREDIT CARDS

ADVANTAGES	DISADVANTAGES
Convenience—Credit cards can save you time and trouble; no searching for an ATM or keeping cash on-hand.	Overuse—Revolving credit makes it easy to spend beyond your means.
Record keeping—Credit card statements can help you track your expenses. Some cards even provide year-end summaries that really help out at tax time.	Paperwork—You'll need to save your receipts and check them against your statement each month. This is a good way to ensure that you haven't been overcharged.
Low-cost loans—You can use revolving credit to save today (eg, at a one-day sale), when available cash is a week away.	High-cost fees—Your purchase will suddenly become much more expensive if you carry a balance or miss a payment.
Instant cash—Cash advances are quick and convenient, putting cash in your hand when you need it.	Unexpected fees—Typically, you'll pay between 2% and 4% just to get the cash advance; also, cash advances usually carry high interest rates.
Perks—From frequent flier miles to discounts on automobiles, there is a program out there for everyone. Many credit card companies offer incentive programs based on the amount of purchases you make.	No free lunch—The high interest rates and annual fees associated with credit cards often outweigh the benefits received. Savings offered by credit cards can often be obtained elsewhere.
Build positive credit—Controlled use of a credit card can help you establish credit for the first time or rebuild credit if you've had problems in the past as long as you stay within your means and pay your bills on time.	Deepening your debt—Consumers are using credit more than ever before. If you charge freely, you may quickly find yourself in over your head—as your balance increases, so do your monthly minimum payments.
Purchase protection—Most credit card companies will handle disputes for you. If a merchant won't take back a defective product, check with your credit card company.	Homework—It's up to you to make sure you receive proper credit for incorrect or fraudulent charges.
Balance surfing—Many credit card companies offer low introductory interest rates. These offers allow you to move balances to lower-rate cards.	Teaser rates—Low introductory rates may be an attractive option, but they last only for a limited time. When the teaser rate expires, the interest rate charged on your balance can jump dramatically.

DISABILITY INSURANCE

Your Health Is Your Wealth

If the time and money spent on medical training was viewed as an investment, the return on that investment would be the future income generated from your ability to perform orthopedic surgery.

What is your income worth? Look at the potential earnings of a 35-year-old orthopedic surgeon earning $250,000. He or she will earn approximately $11,893,853 over the next 30 years of his or her career, assuming a modest 3% compound increase in salary (Table 16-2).

Table 16-2

WHAT IS YOUR INCOME WORTH?

POTENTIAL EARNINGS TO AGE 65 WITH 3% COMPOUND ANNUAL INCREASES

AGE	$50,000	$75,000	$100,000	$150,000	$200,000	$250,000
30	$3,023,104	$4,534,656	$6,046,208	$9,069,312	$12,092,416	$15,115,520
35	$2,378,771	$3,568,156	$4,757,541	$7,136,312	$9,515,083	$11,893,853
40	$1,822,963	$2,734,444	$3,645,926	$5,468,889	$7,291,852	$9,114,816
45	$1.343.519	$2,015,278	$2,687,037	$4,030,556	$5,374,074	$6,717,593
50	$929,946	$1,394,918	$1,859,891	$2,789,837	$3,719,782	$4,649,728
55	$573,194	$859,790	$1,146,387	$1,719,581	$2,292,775	$2,865,969

So, what would happen if that ability was compromised due to an accident or illness? Where would the money come from, and how long could you meet your financial obligations without a paycheck? Having a properly structured disability income insurance policy will make sure that you have the money that you need in the event that you are too sick or hurt to work.

To understand the odds of becoming disabled and the duration of disability, see Tables 16-3 and 16-4.

How Policies Are Offered

Disability insurance can be purchased on an individual or group basis. Group insurance is usually provided by an employer or purchased individually from a sponsoring medical association, such as the American Medical Association (AMA) or American College of Surgeons (ACS).

Although initially low in cost, group policies have several limitations. The association or insurance company can cancel them, rates increase as you get older, and premiums are subject to adjustments based on the claims experience of the group. In addition, group and association contracts often contain restrictive definitions of disability as well as less-generous contract provisions.

How Much Can You Purchase?

Disability insurance companies generally limit the amount of coverage that you can purchase to 60% of your earned income. However, there are special limits available to senior medical students, residents, and fellows. Depending upon the specific insurance company, as of this writing, residents and fellows can qualify to purchase monthly benefits of $3,500 to $5,000, regardless of their actual earned income.

Increased Monthly Benefits

For many years, the maximum benefit available to physicians who performed invasive procedures was limited to $10,000 or $15,000 per month, regardless of their earned incomes. As a result, securing a reasonable amount of disability insurance protection

Table 16-3

THE ODDS OF BECOMING DISABLED

PROBABILITY OF BEING DISABLED FOR 90 DAYS OR MORE BEFORE
REACHING AGE 65 (CHANCES OUT OF 1,000 INDIVIDUALS)

MALE		
AGE	# DISABLED	PERCENTAGE
30	331	33.1%
35	313	31.3%
40	291	29.1%
45	263	26.3%
50	226	22.6%
55	176	17.6%
60	106	10.6%

FEMALE		
AGE	# DISABLED	PERCENTAGE
30	566	56.6%
35	517	51.7%
40	452	45.2%
45	375	37.5%
50	293	29.3%
55	210	21.0%
60	119	11.9%

Source: 1985 Commissioners' Individual Disability Table A

had become a significant challenge for highly compensated physicians. However, several companies will now issue policies with monthly benefits up to $15,000 for orthopedic surgeons as well as participate with other carriers' coverage up to $20,000.

The Cost of Disability Insurance

Premium rates are based on several factors including the insured's age, gender, monthly benefit amount, optional riders selected, the state in which the policy is issued, and the occupational classification assigned to his or her medical specialty by the insurance company. The younger you are when the purchase is made, the lower the cost of the insurance. Therefore, you should purchase a policy as early in your career as possible to lock in lower premium rates. Additionally, most insurance companies also offer "step rate" or "graded" premium rates to allow young professionals to pay lower premiums while they are establishing their careers, enabling them to afford more insurance protection during their initial earning years.

Table 16-4

DURATION OF DISABILITY

AVERAGE DURATION OF LONG-TERM* DISABILITY AT VARIOUS AGES (*LASTING 90 DAYS OR MORE)

AGE	DURATION
25	2 years, 2 months
30	2 years, 8 months
35	3 years, 1 month
40	3 years, 6 months
45	3 years, 11 months
50	4 years, 2 months
55	4 years, 5 months

Source: 1985 Commissioners' Individual Disability Table A

The Cost of Being Female

Although actuarially women are better risks for life insurance compared to men, it is the opposite for disability insurance. As a result, women may pay 50% to 75% more for their policies.

However, many disability insurance carriers offer a "multi-life" discount when several physicians from the same hospital or department purchase individual policies *at the same time* and a letter of endorsement is submitted by the program director, graduate medical education (GME) department, or human resource director. While these programs can produce a savings for men, this strategy allows female physicians to save up to 60% on the cost of their disability insurance.

It is important to note that many teaching hospitals and medical associations have existing programs that you can access—without having to take the time and effort to establish them. You should make sure to ask the insurance agent or financial planner you are dealing with about the availability of these programs.

Look at the Savings Using a Multi-Life or Association Discount

Multi-Life Discount

Dr. Jones, a 30-year-old female orthopedic surgery resident in New York, purchased her policy from a well-known insurance company. Assuming a monthly benefit of $3,500, a 90-day waiting period, benefits payable to age 65, a Residual Disability Rider, and a 3% Cost of Living Adjustment Rider, her fixed annual premium would be $3,055. However, that same policy with a unisex rate and "multi-life" discount would cost $2,056—*an annual savings of $999* or approximately 33% off of the normal female rates. If she kept her policy at the same level to age 65, she would save approximately $35,000. If she invested her annual savings at 6% for the 35-year period, her savings would grow to be in excess of $118,000!

Medical Association Discount

Dr. Smith, a 30-year-old female orthopedic surgery resident in New Jersey, purchased her policy from another well-known insurance company. Assuming a monthly benefit of $3,500, a 90-day waiting period, benefits payable to age 67, a Non-Cancellable Rider, an Own-Occupation Rider, a Residual Disability Rider, and a 3% Cost of Living Adjustment Rider, her fixed annual premium would be $3,174. However, that same policy with an association discount would cost $1,373—*an annual savings of $1,801* or approximately 57% off of the normal female rates. If she kept her policy at the same level to age 65, she would save approximately $63,000. If she invested her annual savings at 6% for the 35-year period, her savings would grow to be in excess of $212,000!

Watch Out for Florida and California

It is not unreasonable to think that most orthopedic surgeons would rather be on the beach than in the operating room. Therefore, claims experience has been extremely poor in these states. As a result, policies are typically 10% to 20% more expensive with less liberal contract provisions. If you are not in Florida or California now but plan on moving or returning to either one of these states after you complete your training, you should purchase your policy before you get there. You will be able to lock into lower premium rates for your initial coverage as well as any future additions that you make to your policy.

What to Look for in a Policy

The renewability provision is one of the main features of an individual disability policy. This provision defines your rights when it comes to keeping your policy in force. If you purchase a policy that is *Non-Cancellable* and *Guaranteed Renewable*, the insurance company cannot cancel your policy, increase your premiums, or change any provisions of your policy—even if the issuing company no longer offers similar policies in the future.

Own-Occupation Definition of Disability

Own-Occupation is the most liberal definition of total disability. A policy with this definition pays benefits if you are disabled and "unable to perform the substantial and material duties of your regular occupation." Therefore, if an accident or sickness prevents you from performing orthopedic surgery, you would be considered totally disabled and eligible to receive full disability benefits.

Beware the agent who tells you that this definition of disability is "no longer available" or that you "don't need it." They may be telling you this because their company no longer offers it and/or they do not have the ability to sell it to you!

This definition of disability is far superior to what is referred to as a modified Own-Occupation definition of disability or "loss of earnings" policy. This is the most prevalent type of policy in the industry today and typically pays benefits if you are "unable to perform the substantial and material duties of your occupation *and you are not working.*" Although benefits are still contingent upon your ability to perform orthopedic surgery, your benefits would be proportionally reduced depending upon the income you earn in another occupation—unless you experience a loss of more than 75% or 80% compared to your pre-disability income.

After all, if the price was comparable (or less expensive), why would you settle for a policy that would penalize you by reducing or eliminating your disability benefits for being smart, motivated, and resourceful enough to transition into a new occupation—and be financially successful at it?

Residual Disability Rider

While Own-Occupation is the most liberal definition of disability, it is not the end all. What happens if your physician states that you can still perform orthopedic surgery but he or she requires that you work fewer days per week, less hours per day, or limits the number of surgeries that you can perform? While the Own-Occupation definition of disability protects your specialty, it does not adequately protect your income. Therefore, a Residual Disability Rider must be added to your policy.

While some orthopedic surgeons believe that they are either "in or out" and "operating or not," the fact is that many, if not most, disability situations are gradual as opposed to immediate. Florida disability insurance attorney John P. Murray notes, "I usually see these doctors tough it out until the point where they are just physically unable to do it anymore." This often creates an issue with the insurance carrier where the claims examiners focus on "what changed" to create the disability that warrants benefits—typically in the total disability analysis. Also, the surgeon typically begins doing more consult or office practice as the physical demands of surgery become too much, and this again creates problems in securing quick recognition of disability.

Murray also says, "in circumstances where a client has not opted for the Residual or Partial Disability Rider, the reason given was that the client either did not understand the benefit of the rider or simply wanted to save money. This ultimately was a bad decision in hindsight for the client."

Generally, to qualify for residual disability benefits, you must experience an income loss of 20% or more compared to your pre-disability earnings. Additionally, if your loss of earnings was greater than 75% or 80%, then 100% of your monthly disability benefit would be paid.

Unfortunately, without this rider, the policy will pay "all or nothing" depending upon your ability to perform your duties as an orthopedic surgeon. This rider is also extremely important if you are totally disabled first and then return to your practice with a limited schedule, or if you never meet the definition of "total" disability found in your policy but experience a substantial loss of income due to an accident or sickness.

Cost of Living Adjustment Rider

A Cost of Living Adjustment (COLA) Rider is designed to help your benefits keep pace with inflation after your disability has lasted for 12 months. This adjustment can be a flat percentage or tied to the Consumer Price Index. Although expensive, this rider can provide significant increases to your monthly benefit if you are disabled early in your career. For example, an orthopedic surgeon who is disabled at age 30 and remains that way until age 65 with a $3,500 monthly benefit, payable after 90 days, would potentially collect a cumulative benefit of $1,459,500. However, with a 3% compounded COLA, the cumulative benefit would increase to $2,528,907—an increase of more than 73%! However, if cutting the cost of coverage is an issue, this might be the first optional rider to consider excluding from your policy, as it can add 15% or more to your premium.

Future Purchase Option Rider

This rider is a must for young physicians. It allows you to apply for additional disability coverage, regardless of your health, as your income rises. Essentially, you are paying for the right to increase your policy's monthly benefit without doing another exam, blood test, urine test, or answering any medical questions. This guarantees that any medical conditions that develop after your original policy's purchase would be fully covered and not subject to new medical underwriting.

For example, assume that Dr. Stevens, an orthopedic surgery resident, purchased an individual disability policy immediately after he started residency. Two years later, he tore his right ACL while skiing and had an ACL reconstruction. Both the preop and postop notes indicated that arthritis was present. As his policy contained a large future increase option rider, any additional coverage purchased under it would cover his knee as if he never had a problem. However, if his policy did not contain a future increase option or if he needed to purchase a new policy, it would most likely exclude any "loss due to disease, disorder, treatment, or complication related to the right knee." Although Dr. Stevens is most likely not concerned about his knee now, he does not know how this might affect his ability to work in the future—especially if the arthritis worsened as he aged. Therefore, you should always purchase a policy with as much future increase option that is available when you are young and healthy.

Why Purchase Your Policy as a Resident or Fellow?

If you graduate and your new employer provides you with long-term disability (LTD) coverage, it will be taken into consideration by the insurance company in determining the maximum amount of individual insurance you can purchase. As a result, in some cases, you may be eligible to purchase less coverage as an attending (making much more money) than you could have purchased under the "beginning professional" special limits offered to residents and fellows.

A Case Study

Dr. Keller will be completing his residency and entering private practice. His starting salary will be $200,000 per year, and his employer will be providing him with disability insurance that covers 60% of his salary with a maximum monthly benefit of $10,000. Therefore, Dr. Keller would collect $10,000 per month in the event of his disability. This insurance is mandatory, and Dr. Keller cannot "waive" the coverage even if he desired.

After reviewing the policy provisions, Dr. Keller becomes aware of the limitations of employer-provided group LTD coverage and decides to purchase an individual policy to supplement the coverage paid by his employer. Using the Issue and Participation limits of a well-known insurance company, Dr. Keller's agent tells him that he can purchase a policy with a monthly benefit of only $2,670.

Dr. Keller is now discouraged, remembering that he could have purchased as much as $5,000 per month as a resident or fellow. In addition to the $5,000 monthly benefit, his policy could have also included the right to purchase up to an additional $10,000 per month, regardless of his health, as his earnings continued to increase. Based upon an initial monthly benefit amount of $2,670, his increase option is now limited to $5,340 (twice the base amount).

Assuming Dr. Keller has no other disability coverage and decides to leave this practice to work for another that provides little or no disability insurance, this can cause a major problem if he is no longer healthy. He may no longer be able to purchase more disability insurance at any price, or any new policies purchased may include an exclusion rider due to subsequent changes in his health.

The moral of the story is that bad things happen to good people, and health, not money, is what buys disability insurance. Money is only the thing that keeps your policy in force. Purchasing disability insurance is like purchasing a parachute. If you go up in a plane with one, and you pull the rip cord in the event of an emergency, it will open every time, and you will land safely. However, if you go up in a plane without a parachute, nobody is going to sell it to you on the way down. Therefore, you need to purchase disability insurance when you "do not need it" to have it when you do need it.

LIFE INSURANCE

A life insurance policy is a contract with an insurance company that will pay your beneficiary a sum of money in the event of your death. Due to its potential to appreciate in value, along with its tax-favored status, it can be used to solve even the most complex financial planning challenges.

Types of Life Insurance

There are many types of life insurance policies available in today's market. However, most policies fall into 1 of 4 categories—term life, whole life, universal life, and variable universal life (Table 16-5).

Term Life

Term life insurance is usually the most appropriate for orthopedic surgery residents and fellows. It allows you to purchase the largest death benefit while minimizing your (initial) premium outlay. Term insurance offers pure protection and does not build cash value.

You should purchase a substantial amount of term insurance when you are young to protect your future insurability. You can always convert your policy to permanent insurance at a later date, regardless of your health, if your policy contains a conversion option.

When you purchase a term policy, you are buying coverage for a specified period of time. If you die within the term of the policy, the insurance company will pay the death benefit to your beneficiary. The majority of term policies purchased today have fixed premium rates for 5, 10, 15, 20, 25, or even 30 years.

Term Conversion Option

A large number of term policies allow you to convert some or all of the death benefit of your term policy to other forms of permanent insurance regardless of your future health. This is an extremely valuable feature for residents and fellows whose incomes and financial situations will change dramatically. Ideally, if your goal is to convert to whole life, you should only purchase your term policy from a company that has a reputation for offering a broad array of competitive whole life insurance policies.

Waiver of Premium Rider

Another important aspect of a life insurance policy is the waiver of premium rider. This rider enables you to have the premiums of the policy paid for by the insurance company in the event of your disability.

While most companies offer the waiver of premium on all types of life insurance, there is no more important application of this rider than with whole life. In addition

Table 16-5

COMPARISON OF TYPES OF LIFE INSURANCE

	TERM LIFE	WHOLE LIFE	UNIVERSAL LIFE	VARIABLE UNIVERSAL LIFE
PREMIUM	Premiums start low, increase at each renewal	Level	Flexible	Flexible
COVERAGE	Usually renewable until at least age 70; for some policies, up to age 95	For life	For life	For life
DEATH BENEFIT	Guaranteed	Guaranteed	May be guaranteed, depending on policy	May be guaranteed, depending on policy
		May increase with dividends	Can be increased or decreased	Can be increased or decreased; varies relative to cash value investment returns
CASH VALUE	None	Guaranteed	Guaranteed minimum interest rate	Not guaranteed
		May increase with dividends	Varies based on interest rates	Fluctuates with underlying investment performance
POLICY LOANS ALLOWED?	Not applicable	Yes	Yes	Yes
		May be able to borrow up to 100% of total cash surrender value less annual loan interest rate	Same as whole life, but usually available at lower net interest rate (ie, pay the interest rate and get a credit back to the policy)	Same as whole life, but usually available at lower net interest rate (ie, pay the interest rate and get a credit back to the policy)
CASH WITHDRAWALS ALLOWED?	Not applicable	No	Yes	Yes
CASH VALUE ACCOUNT GROWTH	No cash value account	Insurance company determines cash value and declares dividends based on performance of its general investment portfolio	Insurance company determines cash value interest crediting rates based on current interest rate returns to the company	Cash value account growth depends upon the investment performance of the subaccounts you choose

to providing for the continuation of life insurance protection, the savings component of the policy is also maintained as 'cash values continue to build. This characteristic provides a unique benefit to the policyholder that cannot be matched by even the best stocks, bonds, or mutual fund investments.

Whole Life

In addition to providing a death benefit, whole life policies build cash value. When you purchase a whole life policy, you traditionally pay a fixed premium for the life of the policy. Part of your premium payments go to the insurance company to cover the cost of the death benefit element of the policy, while the balance is invested in the insurance company's general account.

The cash value of a life insurance policy grows on a tax-deferred basis and can be accessed through policy loans or by surrendering the contract. The level premium structure, guaranteed rate of return, and guaranteed death benefit make whole life an attractive choice for some buyers. Unlike the policies that follow, the only "moving part" in a whole life insurance policy is its dividend.

Whole life offers the ability to provide value in excess of its guarantees through dividends. Dividends are paid to the policyholders if declared by the Board of Directors. When dividends are declared, they have 3 components:

- ✓ The insurance company's investment rate of return in excess of the guaranteed return promised in the policy
- ✓ Mortality experience, which is better than that which is guaranteed in the policy
- ✓ Expenses of policy administration, which are less than the cost guaranteed in the policy

In addition, life insurance is considered an "exempt asset" in many states, including New York, Texas, and Florida—and is specifically protected from the claims of creditors, including malpractice. However, state laws vary widely when it comes to protecting life insurance. As a result, it is important to know whether your state exempts some, all, or none of the cash value in your policy. If you are in a state with an unlimited exemption, besides helping you accumulate wealth, it can play a vital role in your estate and asset protection plan.

Unfortunately, the advantages of whole life insurance have been minimized or often overlooked by the financial services industry. As a result, you may have read or been taught that you should "buy term and invest the difference." This strategy calls for term insurance to be owned for a period of time and then cancelled when your other assets are considered to be "adequate," typically at the start of retirement. What you are not taught is that this strategy simply does not work!

In fact, by properly coordinating and integrating whole life insurance with other assets, you can enjoy increased access, flexibility, and control over your wealth throughout your lifetime. This culminates with retirement options that may otherwise not be available. It is for these reasons that whole life insurance should be the heart of a physician's financial plan.

Universal Life

Universal life was developed in the late 1970s to overcome some of the "disadvantages" of term and whole life insurance. When your premiums are paid, expense, insurance, and maintenance charges are deducted, and the remainder is invested in the insurance company's general account.

Most universal life policies contain a guaranteed minimum interest rate that will be applied to the cash value. Any returns above the guaranteed minimum will vary with the performance of the insurance company's portfolio. Universal life does not allow you to decide how your premiums are invested. However, as the policy owner, you have the ability to vary the amount as well as the frequency of your premium payments. This type of policy is best for someone looking for the flexibility to change his or her premium payments if his or her financial situation changes.

However, if interest rates decline or the insurance company's mortality or expenses increase, the crediting rate on the cash portion of the policy could decrease. This can lead to premium payments that are larger than expected to maintain the policy's death benefit, cause you to reduce the policy's death benefit to allow you to make the same premium payments, or force you to borrow from your cash value to subsidize the premium payments that you are making compared to the premium payments that you should be making. Unfortunately, by coupling increasing insurance costs with a declining interest rate environment, policies can "blow-up" or implode (see more about this under "Variable Universal Life").

Universal Life with a Secondary No-Lapse Guarantee

This policy is very similar to a traditional universal life policy; however, the insurance company guarantees that the death benefit on the policy will remain in effect even if the cash value goes to zero. This is known as a "secondary guarantee." If the policy owner makes premium payments in a timely fashion, the policy's death benefit is guaranteed to the age of 100, or longer.

The advent of this policy can be attributed to the number of policies that did not perform as illustrated or "imploded." Suddenly, what's old is new again.

As a result of the poor state of the economy at the time this was written, some carriers are no longer offering this type of policy.

Variable Universal Life

While whole life insurance provides the policy owner with guaranteed premiums, guaranteed cash values, and a guaranteed death benefit, this is not the case with a variable universal life insurance policy. Generally, premiums for a variable universal life insurance policy are only guaranteed for a limited period of time. There is no guaranteed death benefit, and there is no guaranteed cash value (as the policy owner decides how his or her cash value will be invested, retaining all investment risk). Variable universal life is a flawed life insurance concept in and of itself and, therefore, should almost always be avoided.

THE ROTH IRA: THE GOVERNMENT'S GIFT TO RESIDENTS AND FELLOWS

Although it has been around since 1998 and is one of the best financial tools available to (most) orthopedic surgery residents and fellows, the Roth IRA continues to be underused. Unfortunately, all too often, it is not until after orthopedic surgeons complete their training and no longer qualify do they desire to try to take advantage of the benefits that a Roth IRA provides.

WHAT IS A TRADITIONAL IRA?

A traditional IRA is an individual retirement account that allows you and your spouse to save for retirement by sheltering funds from taxation until they are withdrawn. The maximum amount that may be deducted is restricted, however, if you or your spouse are participating in an employer-sponsored retirement plan. If this is the case, depending on the level of modified adjusted gross income (MAGI), a deduction may be allowed for all, none, or only a portion of an IRA contribution.

If you are covered by an employer-sponsored retirement plan and your MAGI exceeds certain established thresholds, your deduction for your traditional IRA contribution is reduced or eliminated as shown in Table 16-6.

WHAT IS A ROTH IRA?

A Roth IRA is an individual retirement account named after Senator William V. Roth, Jr. (R-Delaware) that allows you and your spouse to make nondeductible contributions to save for retirement. However, rather than growing on a tax-deferred basis, all "qualified" distributions are made on an income tax-free basis. Contributions may be made to both a traditional and Roth IRA in the same year, but are subject to the total annual limits.

A Roth IRA, like a traditional IRA, is not itself an investment, but a tax-advantaged vehicle in which you can hold some of your investments, including, but not limited to, mutual funds, stocks, bonds, futures, options, CDs, or even money market funds. You need to decide how to invest your Roth IRA dollars based on your own tolerance for risk and investment philosophy. How fast your Roth IRA dollars grow is largely a function of the investments you choose to fund the IRA.

For 2009, an individual may contribute the lesser of $5,000 or 100% of compensation for the year to a traditional and/or a Roth IRA. For a married couple, an additional $5,000 may be contributed on behalf of a lesser earning (or nonworking) spouse, using a spousal account. Additionally, if an IRA owner is age 50 or older, he or she may contribute an additional $1,000 ($2,000 if your spouse is also age 50 or older).

As with many tools that offer tax advantages, Congress has limited who can contribute to a Roth IRA based upon income. A taxpayer can only contribute the maximum amount if his or her MAGI is below a certain level. Otherwise, a phase-out of allowed contributions runs throughout the MAGI ranges shown in Table 16-7. Once MAGI hits the top of the range, no contribution is allowed at all.

However, once a Roth IRA is established, the balance in the account remains tax-sheltered, even if the taxpayer's income rises above the threshold. (The thresholds are just for annual eligibility to contribute, not for eligibility to maintain an account.)

WHEN AND TO WHICH SHOULD YOU CONTRIBUTE?

If you want to make a traditional or Roth IRA contribution for the year, you have until the due date of that year's federal income tax return. For most people, this is April 15 of the following year. However, if you contribute to your traditional or Roth IRA after December 31, you should tell the IRA trustee or custodian for which year the contribution is being made. For example, if you make a contribution in February 2010 for the 2009 tax year, you should clearly identify the contribution as being made for the

Table 16-6

IF YOUR FEDERAL INCOME TAX FILING STATUS IS:	YOUR IRA DEDUCTION IS REDUCED IF YOUR MAGI IS BETWEEN:	YOUR DEDUCTION IS ELIMINATED IF YOUR MAGI IS:
Single or head of household	$55,000-$65,000	$65,000 or more
Married filing jointly or qualifying widow(er)	$89,000-$109,000 (combined)	$109,000 or more (combined)
Married filing separately	$0-$10,000	$10,000 or more

Table 16-7

IF YOUR FEDERAL FILING STATUS IS:	YOUR ROTH IRA CONTRIBUTION IS REDUCED IF YOUR MAGI IS:	YOU CANNOT CONTRIBUTE TO A ROTH IRA IF YOUR MAGI IS:
Single or head of household	More than $105,000 but less than $120,000	$120,000 or more
Married filing jointly or qualifying widow(er)	More than $166,000 but less than $176,000	$176,000 or more
Married filing separately	More than $0 but less than $10,000	$10,000 or more

"prior year"—in this case, 2009. Otherwise, the trustee or custodian may assume that the contribution is for 2010 (the year in which it is received) and report it as such.

Also note that the contribution deadline is not extended by any extension you may receive to file your income tax return. Therefore, if you obtain an automatic 4-month extension, while you may have additional time to file your tax return, you don't have any additional time to make a traditional or Roth IRA contribution.

If you are like me and believe taxes will be higher in the future than they are now, you should probably consider a Roth IRA compared to a traditional IRA.

If we look at the history of income taxes from 1913-2006, the average highest marginal individual income tax rate is 60.3% (Figure 16-1).

With the "war on terror," aging "baby boomers" drawing on Social Security benefits, endless bailout plans, an increasing deficit, and a host of other factors, what do you think is going to happen to tax rates in the future? If you are a skeptic like me, you would probably rather pay taxes today to have the ability to pay less in taxes during your retirement.

So why defer income when your tax bracket is low to pay taxes when your bracket is high? Isn't that "reverse tax planning?"

Therefore, orthopedic surgery residents and fellows should look to take advantage of the Roth IRA while it is available to them based on their incomes.

WITHDRAWING YOUR MONEY

A withdrawal from a Roth IRA (including both contributions and investment earnings) is completely tax free (and penalty free) if made at least 5 years after you first establish any Roth IRA and if one of the following also applies:

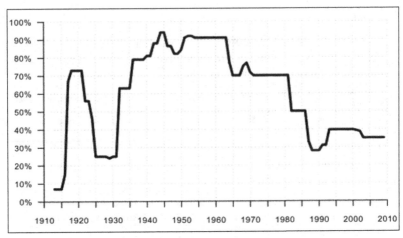

Figure 16-1. Top U.S. Federal marginal income tax rate from 1913 to 2009.

- ✓ You have reached age 59½ by the time of the withdrawal
- ✓ The withdrawal is made due to qualifying disability
- ✓ The withdrawal is made for first-time homebuyer expenses ($10,000 lifetime limit)
- ✓ The withdrawal is made by your beneficiary or estate after your death

Withdrawals that meet these conditions are referred to as "qualified distributions." If the above conditions aren't met, any portion of a withdrawal that represents investment earnings will be subject to federal income tax and may also be subject to a 10% premature distribution tax if you are under age 59½.

ROTH IRA STRENGTHS

Unlike traditional IRAs, you can contribute to a Roth IRA for every year that you have taxable compensation, including the year in which you reach age 70½ and every year thereafter.

The IRS requires you to take annual required minimum distributions from traditional IRAs beginning when you reach age 70½. These withdrawals are calculated to dispose of all of the money in the traditional IRA over a given period of time. Roth IRAs are not subject to the required minimum distribution (RMD) rule. In fact, you are not required to take a single distribution from a Roth IRA during your life (although distributions are generally required after your death). This can be a significant advantage in terms of your estate planning.

You can even contribute to a Roth IRA if you are covered by an employer-sponsored retirement plan. Unlike a traditional IRA where you make deductible contributions, your ability to contribute to a Roth IRA (or to make nondeductible contributions to a traditional IRA) does not depend on whether you or your spouse is covered by an employer-sponsored retirement plan. The fact that one of you is covered by such a plan has no bearing on your allowable contribution to a Roth IRA.

Finally, like a traditional IRA, you do not have to make a contribution to your Roth IRA for any year unless you choose to. Within the limits on the amount that you can contribute each year, you can exercise complete discretion in deciding how much and when to save.

THE LAST WORD ON ROTH IRAS

As Roth IRAs tend to favor younger taxpayers who have a long period until retirement and those who expect to be in a higher tax bracket in the future when funds are withdrawn, they should be one of the first financial planning strategies implemented by surgeons.

Remember that an IRA is not itself an investment, but a tax-advantaged vehicle in which you can hold some of your investments. Choosing specific investments to fund your IRA is an important decision and should be an overall part of an integrated and coordinated financial plan.

If you do not have the time, energy, or inclination to do this yourself, retain a qualified financial services professional. He or she will analyze your situation and help you select investments that are appropriate for your goals, risk tolerance, and time horizon.

CONCLUSION

When you dreamed of becoming a doctor, you knew that the process would require hard work, dedication, and a tremendous time commitment, yet nothing could stop you from achieving that goal.

So why is it that so many orthopedic surgeons don't "plan to fail" but simply "fail to plan" when it comes to their personal finances and the business of medicine? Perhaps one of my clients said it best when he told me "if you don't have the interest, you don't have the time" but "if you have the interest, you find the time!"

Hopefully, after reading this chapter, you have a better understanding of the financial planning issues that you face during residency and now have a better ability to make well-informed, educated decisions regarding the management of credit card debt, the purchase of disability and life insurance, and the reasons why you might want to consider establishing a Roth IRA at this stage of your career.

GLOSSARY OF TERMS

Cost of Living Adjustment (COLA) Rider: Rider found in a disability policy designed to keep your disability benefits in pace with inflation after you have collected benefits for 12 months.

Dividends: Amount of earnings paid out after the company sets aside funds required to cover contractual obligations (reserves), operating expenses, contingencies, and general business purposes. Typically found in whole life insurance policies.

Emergency Fund: Money set aside for unexpected financial situations. Most financial experts recommend saving 3 to 6 months of income in an easily liquidated account such as a checking, savings, or money market account.

Future Increase Option Rider: Rider found in a disability policy that allows you to increase your coverage, regardless of your health, as your income rises. This is subject to your income and other disability insurance in force.

Guaranteed Renewable Disability Insurance: A disability policy that cannot be cancelled nor have its terms, other than premium rates, changed by the insurance company. Premiums may only be changed by class and may be subject to approval by the appropriate regulatory agency.

Individual Retirement Account (IRA): A retirement account that provides either a tax-deferred or tax-free way of saving for retirement. Traditional and Roth IRAs are the most common.

Insurability: The ability to be insured. Meeting the conditions under which an insurance company will issue insurance to an applicant (based on standards set by the insurance company).

Level Premium Term Life Insurance: A life insurance policy in which the premium rates remain the same for the duration of the contract. Typically, premiums for this type of policy will be higher in the early years but lower in later years compared to term life insurance policies that have increasing premium rates.

Life Insurance Policy: A contract with an insurance company that will pay your beneficiary a sum of money in the event of your death.

Modified Adjusted Gross Income (MAGI): Used to determine how much can be contributed to certain personal retirement programs. MAGI is adjusted gross income (AGI), modified by various adjustments.

Non-Cancellable Guaranteed Renewable Disability Insurance: A disability policy where the premium rates and provisions are guaranteed once the policy is issued—typically to age 65 or 67.

Own-Occupation Definition of Disability: Definition found in a disability policy that pays benefits if you are unable to perform your duties as an orthopedic surgeon—even if you are earning the same or more money in another occupation or medical specialty.

Permanent Insurance: An umbrella term for life insurance policies that do not expire (unlike term life insurance) and combine a death benefit with a savings portion or cash value.

Residual Disability Rider: Rider found in a disability policy that pays benefits proportionate to your loss of income in the event you are still able to work in your occupation but are experiencing a loss of income as you are working fewer hours, seeing fewer patients, or doing fewer cases.

Required Minimum Distributions (RMDs): The amount that traditional, SEP, and SIMPLE IRA owners and qualified plan participants must begin withdrawing from their retirement accounts by April 1 following the year they reach age 70½. RMD amounts must then be distributed each subsequent year.

Tax-Deferred Growth: An investment in which some or all taxes are paid at a future date, rather than in the year the investment produces income.

Tax-Free Growth: An investment whose growth is exempt from tax. A Roth IRA is a good example of a vehicle with tax-free growth.

Section III

FELLOWSHIPS: GETTING A POSITION AND SUCCEEDING

Choosing to do a postgraduate fellowship is a weighty decision. You have already spent a long time in college, medical school, and residency, and the thought of prolonging your training one more year may be unpalatable. Then again, maybe the thought of being out on your own is a little frightening also. There are many reasons to do a fellowship and many reasons not to—it all depends on what you want to do once you have finished your training.

What do you need to do to get a top fellowship? A strong residency performance is the cornerstone of obtaining a good fellowship. Beyond that, establishing and maintaining good relationships with select personnel at your institution—among them, ideally, your chairperson and the chief of your institution's orthopedic service corresponding to your fellowship's subspecialty—provides a strong basis for good recommendations. It is also important to have a good research record. Programs prefer candidates who have been motivated to publish during their residencies.

Once you have made a commitment to serving a fellowship, ask yourself exactly what you intend to accomplish during this year of specialty training. The primary goal of most fellowship applicants is to acquire advanced surgical skills, with a secondary aim of improving marketability to both prospective employers and patients. Others seek out a fellowship to bolster their knowledge in an area where they feel their residency training was incomplete.

You can also use fellowship training to strengthen your academic credentials through participation in research projects. If this is important, you will want to determine the nature and strength of the research conducted at each program: Do these types of studies match your interests? Conduct a literature search on the names of the surgeons in the program. What are their specific research interests? How productive have they been? Find out how the institution archives patient records. Have they maintained a computerized database of cases, or will you be sifting through a surgical log to find cases of interest? Is support staff available, such as an epidemiologist or biostatistician, to assist you in study design and manuscript preparation?

Laith M. Jazrawi, MD; Lava Y. Patel, BA; Craig J. Della Valle, MD; Kenneth A. Egol, MD; Steve K. Lee, MD; Brett Young, MD; and Afshin Eli Razi, MD

L. M. Jazrawi, K. A. Egol, & J. D. Zuckerman.
Orthopedic Residency & Fellowship: A Guide to Success (pp. 113-126)
© 2010 Taylor & Francis Group.

If you ultimately plan to seek a faculty position at a teaching hospital, consider the academic reputation of the surgeons with whom you will be working. Fellowship directors with strong academic records are usually active in national organizations. You can easily identify these people at meetings such as those sponsored by the American Academy of Orthopaedic Surgeons (AAOS).

Once you have decided on a specialty, you are ready to assemble a list of programs in that area. A good place to start is by consulting *Postgraduate Orthopaedic Fellowships*, published annually by the AAOS (6300 North River Road, Rosemont, IL 60018, [847] 823-7186, [800] 346-2267; www.aaos.org). One way to assess these programs' relative strengths is to find out the percentage of cases that involve the complex procedures in which you want to gain proficiency. Get hard numbers—and confirm that fellows scrub on those cases. At the same time, be aware that in certain fellowships (eg, in a sports medicine department that covers a professional sports team), your involvement in some areas will of necessity be more "observational."

In some programs, you will be working primarily with one surgeon. In other programs, you will be working with several. Working with a single surgeon makes it easier to develop a one-on-one relationship with him or her. On the other hand, working with several surgeons makes it more likely that you will be exposed to a variety of operative techniques and practice styles.

Fellowships also vary by degree of resident involvement in cases. If residents are not involved, there will be no "competition" for cases; on the other hand, you will more likely be directly responsible for postoperative patient care.

Geographic location is another consideration. Keep in mind that there are several excellent fellowships in Canada and Europe. One resource for learning about these programs is the AAOS Web site.

THE APPLICATION PROCESS

Request fellowship applications no later than July of the beginning of your fourth post-graduate year (PGY-4). At the same time, request letters of recommendation so that they will be available by the fall. Most programs require 2 or 3 letters, including a letter from the chairperson of your residency program. It is conventional to provide letter writers with your curriculum vitae (CV), your personal statement, and a list of programs to which you are applying.

Applications range anywhere from a 1-page form to a several-page document requesting reams of seemingly irrelevant information; fellowship programs in some specialties have agreed on a common ("universal") application. Once you have an application in hand, fill it out carefully, and return it quickly; the earlier you do so, the better your chances of being offered an interview. Many programs—particularly those that do not participate in a match—review and act upon applications as soon as they are received. You might consider using Omniform (www.scansoft.com) software that allows you to scan in your applications, fill them out, and print them.

Most programs require a CV and a personal statement. Use your personal statement to explain why you are interested in the discipline, what your specific goals are for the fellowship, and what your plans are upon completion of the fellowship. Keep the personal statement brief and to the point; your readers will appreciate it.

THE FELLOWSHIP MATCH

The matching program is designed to maximize every applicant's chances of being accepted by the fellowship program of his or her choice. Fellowship programs in sports medicine, pediatric orthopedics, foot and ankle, orthopedic trauma, adult reconstructive hip and knee/musculoskeletal oncology, and spine surgery participate in the San Francisco Match Program (SF Match). Instructions for registering for the match can be found at www.sfmatch.org. Some of these fellowships also use the Centralized Application Service (CAS). The CAS distributes applications to some fellowship training programs. All you have to do is fill out one universal application form, gather one copy of each of the appropriate documents, and mail your entire package to CAS. They process, scan, and distribute your applications to each of the programs that you request. You can access the CAS on the SF Match site under the participating fellowships. For example, for those applying to orthopedic trauma, you can visit http://sfmatch.org/fellowship/f_ota/index.htm.

Fellowship programs in hand surgery participate in the Combined Musculoskeletal Matching Program via the National Residency Match Program (NRMP). Register for the match by calling the NRMP at (202) 828-0566. (More information regarding applications and deadlines is available at www.nrmp.org/fellow/index.html.)

While most programs honor the spirit of the match by refraining from asking you where you intend to rank them, if they do ask you and they are your top choice, by all means, tell them so—it can do nothing but improve your chances of matching there. Of course, only do this if they are indeed your first choice; you do not want to begin your career by alienating future colleagues in your subspecialty.

By the same token, do not include on your rank list any program where you do not want to end up. Once you have finished all of your interviews, go back through your list of programs and review the notes you took after each. (For more on interviews, see Chapter 6 in Section I.) Assess each interview in light of the most important factors you initially established. Now, put it all together with whatever "gestalt" you felt about the program and rank the programs.

THE SPORTS MEDICINE FELLOWSHIP

Many people mistakenly believe that all sports medicine physicians only do arthroscopy. While this is true for a few surgeons, most fellowship-trained sports medicine orthopedists take care of a wide array of athletic injuries to the elbow, shoulder, knee, and ankle in athletes, weekend warriors, and non-athletes requiring arthroscopic as well as open treatment. Sports medicine fellowships provide exposure to treatment of sports-related injuries through field experience and team coverage, operative experience, clinics, and research. Programs vary in their representation of each of these 4 experiences.

WHAT TO LOOK FOR IN A SPORTS MEDICINE FELLOWSHIP

Field Experience and Team Coverage

Team coverage during your fellowship can provide invaluable experience in the care and management of sports teams and on-field evaluation of sports injuries. Often a unique facet of this experience is the opportunity to interact with trainers, who offer a different perspective on the care of athletes. Some fellowships cover professional teams, while others are limited to high school or college teams; the latter, while less prestigious, usually involves a more active role for the fellow. A disadvantage of professional team coverage is that fellows tend to be relegated to observational roles; still, if your ultimate aim is to cover professional teams, such a fellowship is critical.

Operative Experience

Most programs offer adequate exposure to shoulder and knee cases; exposure to elbow, wrist/hand, and ankle/foot cases is more variable. Ask to see a list of cases from the previous month or year to determine whether the fellowship you are investigating provides an adequate caseload of the procedures you are most interested in. Annual caseload varies greatly among programs. Some programs can expose the fellow to approximately 250 cases per year, while others boast of upward of 500. When interviewing, be sure to ask the fellows whether they spend most of their time in the operating room actively performing cases or observing. Although it is nice to see a variety of cases, some fellows may feel more comfortable with a more hands-on experience. Program size and attending interaction is also important.

Clinic Experience

Time spent with attendings in the office or clinic can be very rewarding. In these settings, you can learn about the non-operative management of athletic injuries, physical and occupational therapy protocols, and operative indications, as well as improve your physical examination and diagnostic skills. Fellowships vary greatly in the fellow involvement in office hours and clinic time, so it is prudent to investigate this aspect of the experience carefully.

Research

Most fellowships require at least one project to be completed and submitted for publication. If you are not interested in pursuing research, look for programs with minimal research requirements. For those interested in pursuing research, seek out programs that have traditionally produced quality research, have adequate research facilities, and are appropriately staffed to conduct meaningful research. What is the track record of the research faculty? How easy is it for fellows to start a project? Does the fellowship include financial support for new projects?

Finally, it is important to consider how well a given fellowship program complements your residency experience. For example, if your residency was top-heavy with open shoulder procedures, you may prefer a fellowship program where all or at least most shoulder cases are treated arthroscopically.

APPLYING FOR A SPORTS MEDICINE FELLOWSHIP

In 2008, Arthroscopy Association of North America (AANA) and American Orthopaedic Society for Sports Medicine (AOSSM) created a joint effort to re-establish a match process for sports medicine fellowships. The actual match process is now being administered through the SF Match. The majority of programs have agreed to cooperate and participate in SF Match, and it currently includes 92 programs representing 219 fellowship positions participating. The SF Match site can be viewed by visiting www.sfmatch.org.

You should access/request applications in July of the beginning of your PGY-4 year. The SF Match CAS can be accessed by visiting http://sfmatch.org/fellowship/f_sports/index.htm. For general information regarding the application process, please visit www.sportsmed.org/tabs/Index.aspx and click on the "Fellowships" tab.

Sports medicine fellowships are among the most popular and competitive in orthopedics. To maximize your chances of obtaining a good fellowship, get involved in research—preferably in sports medicine—and foster a relationship with your sports medicine faculty. Most programs require a fellowship research project and naturally prefer candidates who have already done some. Moreover, the topic of your research provides a nice introduction for your interview—especially if the fellowship director has similar interests.

Though any publications will certainly weigh heavily in your favor, if they are not sports-related, few interviewers will ask about them. Last, as it is such a competitive field, a call made on your behalf can be very influential. Cultivate relationships with faculty members involved in the academic community, especially those who know fellowship directors.

Programs that work outside of the match pose a problem. They offer applicants spots prior to the match, and unless one of these is your first choice, you may not want to commit to it. The dilemma is that the match is so competitive that giving up such a position and then not matching results in you ending up holding the bag. You thus need to get a feeling of how competitive you are in the match ahead of time. This can be accomplished by your residency director calling your match programs. If you are at risk for not matching, taking a program outside of the match may be wise.

Despite all of your best intentions and hard work, you may not be granted interviews at the programs you are most interested in or even match at all. There is still hope. Fellowships do not always fill all of their positions, and something may open up after the match.

THE ADULT RECONSTRUCTION FELLOWSHIP
WHAT TO LOOK FOR IN AN ADULT RECONSTRUCTIVE FELLOWSHIP

The primary goal of most applicants for an adult reconstructive fellowship is to gain advanced experience in complex primary and revision total joint arthroplasty of the hip and knee. As the population of patients with total joint implants increases in number and grows older, the number of them requiring revision surgery is ever-increasing, in turn calling for an even greater number of surgeons trained in performing these difficult procedures. In considering fellowship programs, determine what percentage of cases performed are in fact complex revision procedures. Ask to see specific numbers and make sure that you will be exposed to the complex cases that will add the most to your experience. Although some centers perform a large number of arthroplasties, they may be mostly primary reconstructions.

It is also important to ensure that you spend time in the office as issues regarding preoperative planning and patient management will be learned. Spending every day in the operating room is unnecessary for the majority of graduating residents, and spending time in the office is an important part of an advanced training experience. You will also learn important aspects of running an office, billing, and general patient management that you will otherwise not be exposed to while in the operating room. Research experience is another factor to be considered, particularly if you are interested in an academic career in the future. In particular, look for mentors with a strong track record of publication and an interest in training future leaders in the field.

Another consideration is the types of procedures you want to become more familiar with during your fellowship. Although the majority of fellowships concentrate on hip and knee arthroplasty, some fellowships will expose you to upper extremity arthroplasty and complex osteotomy procedures, such as periacetabular osteotomies. As knowledge and interest in femoroacetabular impingement (FAI) has also increased, some fellowships will provide exposure to procedures aimed at correcting these anatomic abnormalities, such as open surgical dislocations and hip arthroscopy. Find out whether the institution at which you may train performs an adequate volume of these specific procedures. In addition, make sure that you will not be "competing" with other fellows (such as a shoulder fellow if you are interested in learning more about shoulder arthroplasty or the sports fellow if you are interested in hip arthroscopy) for these cases. Similarly, some fellowship programs provide significant exposure to knee ligament reconstructions, cartilage resurfacing procedures, and other sports-medicine-related surgeries. Fellowships also exist that combine an adult reconstructive experience with significant exposure to pelvic and acetabular trauma.

APPLYING FOR AN ADULT RECONSTRUCTIVE FELLOWSHIP

A match has recently been organized for adult reconstructive fellowships. Go to www.aahks.org for more information regarding the match including deadlines and a universal application. This will allow you to interview at multiple programs and "levels the playing field," optimizing your chances at training at the fellowship of your choice.

THE HAND FELLOWSHIP

The field of hand surgery is very broad. Hand surgeons treat many different types of problems in a diverse patient population. Your fellowship will train you in joint arthroplasty, fracture and dislocation treatment, ligament reconstruction, microvascular surgery including replantation surgery and free tissue transfers, arthroscopy, tendon repair, peripheral nerve procedures, congenital deformity, arthritis procedures, and oncology. Many hand-trained surgeons also choose to manage the entire upper extremity and include shoulder and elbow disorders in their practice.

In addition to intellectual interest in the field, other factors may be important to you in choosing a fellowship. Do you want a practice with mostly outpatient procedures (hand and sports)? Do you want to treat acute trauma patients (hand, spine, and trauma)? Are you looking for a field that will make you more marketable when looking for a position? Do some soul searching to figure out what you want to be doing in 10 years and how you want to get there.

WHAT TO LOOK FOR IN A HAND FELLOWSHIP

Most hand fellowship programs are small, with only 1 to 3 fellows and 4 to 6 attendings. If you are unhappy with your fellowship choice, both you and the program will suffer. You want to ensure that you not only get along with the attendings, but also develop relationships with them that will both enhance your learning during your fellowship and provide you with friends and colleagues for years to come. A hand fellowship is just the start of a lifelong relationship with your mentors and institution. The academic world of hand surgery is a small place. For the rest of your career, you will continually see the same people you interviewed with (both fellow applicants and attendings) at local and national meetings.

A good place to start looking at the fellowship programs, as mentioned previously, is *Postgraduate Orthopaedic Fellowships*, published annually by AAOS. In the 2009 edition, 55 hand fellowships were listed. These fellowships are all accredited by the Accreditation Council for Graduate Medical Education (ACGME), which means that you will be qualified to take the Certificate of Added Qualification (CAQ) examination in hand surgery upon completion of your fellowship. Beware of fellowships billing themselves as "upper extremity with a significant amount of hand"—if they aren't ACGME-accredited, you won't be able to become board certified in hand surgery. You must have your CAQ to be a member of the main hand surgery society in the US—the American Society for Surgery of the Hand (ASSH).

While most programs will expose fellows to all facets of hand surgery, most programs emphasize one area or another. Among the most important aspects of selecting a hand surgery fellowship is finding one with an emphasis that matches your interests. For instance, you may or may not want a fellowship that has a lot of shoulder and elbow surgery.

Hand surgery is a regional specialty with the majority of surgeons having initial training in either orthopedic or plastic surgery. Find out whether the faculty is predominately orthopedic surgery-based, plastic surgery-based, or a combination of the two (it may have an effect on the type of training or the strengths of teaching that you receive).

APPLYING FOR A HAND FELLOWSHIP

Some hand fellowship programs use a custom application, while others use a universal application. You can find and download the "Universal Hand Surgery Fellowship Application" at www.assh.org/Professionals/Education/ResidentsandFellows/Pages/FellowshipPrograms.aspx. This site can also be used to find information on participating programs.

Most programs participate in the NRMP via the Combined Musculoskeletal Match Program (CMMP). To enroll, obtain an NRMP applicant code (see "The Fellowship Match"). For more information regarding the process and a schedule of dates, please visit www.nrmp.org/fellow/match_name/cmmp/dates.html.

Most programs interview between February and April. As some programs only have 1 interview date, others 2 or 3, and some more than 10, anticipate conflicts between interview dates. Of course, it is always good to have too many interview offers than too few.

Guidelines for fellowship interviews are the same as those for residency (see Chapter 6). Interview day is your chance to talk with attendings and current fellows about the nuts and bolts of the program. Remember the list you made of what you are looking for in a fellowship? This is your opportunity to find out if you will be happy spending a year at the program. Commonly asked questions are the number of cases the fellows did, the breakdown of those cases (how many shoulder, elbow, microvascular, trauma, arthroscopy, congenital, trauma, etc?), fellows' relationships with the attendings (are you treated as a colleague, or as someone to make more money for their practice?), fellows' responsibilities (research, lectures, etc), interactions with the resident staff, the call schedule, and the amount of didactics. Above all, try to get a feel for how happy you will be spending a year and the rest of your career with the person with whom you are interviewing.

Prepare for your interview by doing research about the attendings before you arrive, reviewing the information about the program they sent you, and re-reviewing your CV and personal statement. You want to maximize the brief amount of time you have during each interview and avoid asking questions that are clearly answered in the program's informational packet. Expect to be asked about any research you have done or case reports you have written, and prepare accordingly.

After the interview, be sure to write down all of the details you found out. When it comes time to make your rank list, you will be glad that you did. It is also a good idea to send a thank-you letter to the program for interviewing you. This should be done as soon as possible after the interview and certainly within a week or two.

THE SHOULDER AND ELBOW FELLOWSHIP

Fellowships in shoulder and elbow surgery are relatively new, but their popularity is increasing and the number of fellowships available is increasing. Because there is no accreditation agency for shoulder fellowships, a wide variety of educational opportunities exist, each of which will be more appealing to some individuals than to others. American Shoulder and Elbow Surgeons (ASES) maintains a list of fellowship programs that participate in the Shoulder and Elbow Fellowship match program. This list represents the vast majority of shoulder and elbow fellowships, but there are a few that do not participate in this match, so you will have to do some digging around. Some programs in adult reconstructive orthopedics, most of which are accredited by the ACGME, emphasize shoulder reconstruction.

WHAT TO LOOK FOR IN A SHOULDER AND ELBOW FELLOWSHIP

You can acquire advanced understanding of disorders of the shoulder and elbow in certain sports medicine fellowships as well as upper extremity fellowships. These programs usually include one or more attendings who devote a significant portion of their practice to the shoulder or elbow. It is also important to understand the difference between a sports medicine-oriented physician, who will tend to be treating a relatively young population, and an upper extremity-oriented physician, who will see a larger proportion of hand disorders.

You can also participate in programs that specifically bill themselves as shoulder and elbow fellowships. Because this fellowship category is not governed by ACGME, there is a wide variety of fellowship experiences. Some fellowships concentrate on open surgical techniques and others on arthroscopic techniques. Some have more or less elbow exposure. A program that concentrates on trauma, with minimal sports medicine, will probably provide you with lots of experience with shoulder fractures and hemiarthroplasties but little with labral tears and total shoulder arthroplasty; other shoulder fellowships will have strong arthroplasty and arthroscopy emphases, with minimal trauma. Select the fellowship most appropriate for you (ie, one that will complement your residency experience and prepare you for your envisioned career).

As in other subspecialties, some fellowships may be structured as a "mentorship," where the fellow works primarily with a single surgeon, or the fellowship may involve experience with several surgeons, all of whom may approach the same problems differently.

Last, when evaluating a prospective shoulder fellowship, consider the fellowship director. What are the director's academic strengths? What kind of personality does he or she have? At what level are his or her teaching skills and "political" influence? Remember that, if only because of the numbers, fellows are usually closer to their program's director than are residents.

APPLYING FOR A SHOULDER FELLOWSHIP

The most common way orthopedic surgery residents apply for a shoulder and elbow fellowship is through the coordinated match program sponsored by the ASES. The ASES Web site (www.ases-assn.org) contains a list of all of the shoulder and elbow fellowship programs that participate in the match. Typically, the deadline for application is late summer or early fall of each year, with interviews performed during the fall. The match works similarly to residency, with each applicant ranking his or her programs in order of preference and each fellowship program ranking the applicants in order of preference. For a list of ACGME-accredited shoulder and elbow fellowship programs, please see Appendix H.

THE ORTHOPEDIC TRAUMA FELLOWSHIP

The decision to pursue a fellowship in orthopedic trauma, as with any other fellowship, must be made carefully. Most trauma fellowships are physically demanding with significant on-call time, which, by the nature of the subspecialty, is typically quite busy. A trauma fellowship, because it provides advanced operative training in all areas of the body, may be useful for those pursuing careers in other areas of reconstructive orthopedics.

WHAT TO LOOK FOR IN AN ORTHOPEDIC TRAUMA FELLOWSHIP

Fellowships in orthopedic trauma offer advanced training in the treatment of fractures and their sequelae. They typically include exposure to large volumes of polytrauma patients and complex intra-articular fractures, as well as pelvic and acetabular fractures, nonunions, malunions, and post-traumatic osteomyelitis. Several trauma fellowships also include exposure to spinal trauma. The majority of fellowships are at major regional trauma centers. A few are based at tertiary referral centers, where the experience is more heavily weighted toward definitive fixation and reconstruction than toward acute management.

Talking to current fellows is particularly important in judging whether a particular program is suited to your needs. Determine the amount of operative time and clinic time you would have as a fellow, as well as teaching, autonomy, and research time. Issues do arise between residents and fellows in determining who has priority in the operating room; this of course should be divided into level-appropriate cases. Talking with the residents as well as the fellows should give you an idea as to the nature of this dynamic.

While most trauma fellowships offer significant experience in treating long-bone fractures, an applicant needs to evaluate the number of complex cases being done, such as pelvis and acetabulum fractures. Additionally, many fellowships offer experience in complex reconstructive techniques such as Ilizarov external fixation technique, complex foot procedures, and pelvic osteotomies. Spine trauma care is offered at some programs; at most places, however, this is performed by the spine service, not the trauma service. Make sure that the programs you are applying to fit with your interests, as the experiences offered at different institutions vary greatly.

Call schedules range from every other to about every fifth night, with some programs requiring a fellow to be in-house (often this is not an issue, as cases frequently go all night). In some programs, fellows initially take call with an attending and subsequently function as a junior attending with senior attending backup. Some programs require fellows to take attending-level call at outside institutions, which may not be major trauma centers; this may add little to your training and take up valuable time. It is also worthwhile to inquire about the quality and role of the house staff at the institution as these significantly affect the quality of life for the fellow.

Research opportunities can be another important factor to consider when choosing a trauma fellowship. While most programs have active clinical research programs, not all have basic science opportunities. In addition, there may not be time protected for research activity. Research productivity may be important in finding a position after fellowship, particularly in the academic sector.

Most orthopedic trauma fellowships offer excellent training in trauma surgery. Different philosophies and protocols exist at different institutions, most of which are effective in treating patients. It is important to identify a program where you would be comfortable: the right people, the right cases, the right volume, the right location, and the right lifestyle.

APPLYING FOR AN ORTHOPEDIC TRAUMA FELLOWSHIP

The Fellowship Match for Orthopedic Trauma (OT Match) was established in 2008. It participates in the SF Match (www.sfmatch.org) and uses the CAS. The Orthopaedic Trauma Association (OTA) sponsors the Match and provides general information regarding the process, which can be found at www.ota.org.

Request application materials in July at the beginning of your PGY-4 year. Applications tend to be simple: a CV, several letters of recommendation, and a personal statement are generally all that are required. Interviews are typically conducted between December and February. The problem lies in that offers are often made shortly after the interview session, and the program directors request a quick decision, usually within a day. You may thus feel pressured into accepting an offer from a program before interviewing at your top choice.

The interview process is typically informal. While trauma fellowships are becoming more competitive, they are not yet at the level of those in sports medicine or hand surgery. Interviews usually involve group information sessions and meeting with the program directors and staff, as well as current fellows and residents at the program. Several include rounding with the orthopedic trauma team and/or reviewing the x-ray boards for inpatients. Visiting a program is also the time to evaluate the diversity of cases and whether they meet your interests.

THE PEDIATRIC ORTHOPEDICS FELLOWSHIP

Programs offering pediatric orthopedic fellowships are listed in *Postgraduate Orthopedic Fellowships* (published yearly by the AAOS), which includes important information on the fellowships with brief descriptions of each and indicates which are accredited by the ACGME and which participate in the NRMP—although it is not entirely accurate in this last regard. Not everyone agrees accreditation is needed to get quality training; more information on the value of accreditation can be obtained from your director or chairperson.

WHAT TO LOOK FOR IN A PEDIATRIC ORTHOPEDIC FELLOWSHIP

Know what type of practice you want in the future because pediatric orthopedic fellowships vary greatly. Consider whether you want to work in an academic environment or private practice when your training is finished. Someone working in private practice would not be expected to see the types of cases seen at a major referral center. If you have a special interest (eg, spine, limb deformity correction, or cerebral palsy), look for a program that gives more exposure in those areas.

On-call schedules vary from none to every second or third night. Most are backing up a resident, but you might be required to perform surgery. There might be an attending present or you may be acting as a junior attending with senior attending backup.

Some fellowships are funded through an endowment, while others rely on billing for the surgery you do while on call for some or all of their funding.

All programs require you to write a manuscript suitable for publication or presentation at a national meeting. The number of projects required varies from program to program. Some institutions archive decades' worth of patient records and radiographs, while others are not so organized. Important questions to ask regarding research opportunities include the following: Are personnel available to help me collect data? Do you maintain a database of cases, or will I have to go through OR logs to find what I need? Is there help available for preparing a manuscript?

APPLYING FOR A PEDIATRIC ORTHOPEDIC FELLOWSHIP

The Pediatric Orthopaedic Surgery Fellowship Match (POSM) was established in 2009. The SF Match, described earlier in the chapter, is the specialty match for pediatric orthopedics. The Match takes place in April and will be used to process all applicants who want to start their fellowship training in August of the following year. Please visit www.sfmatch.org for more information. You can also find general information regarding the process at www.posna.org/careers/fellowships/fellowships.asp.

Call programs you are interested in to find out whether they participate in the match, as this changes every year. The safest thing is to start program inquiries at the beginning of your PGY-4 year in July. Remember, programs will be adjusting their interview schedule because it appears that the Match will not be used in the near future. Try to interview by November or December at programs that mean the most to you.

The CAS application service provides the application form for pediatric orthopedic fellowships. It can be accessed and downloaded from the SF Match Web site. Some applications require more documentation than others; keep in mind that it can take 3 to 4 weeks for medical school records or Board scores to be mailed. Most applications require a letter from your program chairperson plus 2 or 3 letters of recommendation, a personal statement, and a CV.

Before the interview, do some research into the institution and the people who will be interviewing you. Many children's hospitals now maintain Web sites, and these can be informative. Perform a literature search of faculty you will be meeting. Many orthopedists in the field have an area of special interest, and it helps for you to be familiar with their work in it. The interview consists of several parts and usually lasts most of the day. Meetings with staff are in both formal and informal settings; you may spend time in clinic, on rounds, or observing in the operating room. Ask to see previous years' breakdown of cases, or at least the previous month's statistics. Speak to current fellows about their experience and the quality of life in the area.

Take notes after the interview. Details and names are easily forgotten after interviewing at a number of programs and meeting dozens of people. Send thank you letters within a week of all interviews and tailor them to express how interested you are in their program. It is also a good idea to follow up the thank you letter with a phone call from your program director to a program if it is your top choice.

THE SPINE FELLOWSHIP

WHAT TO LOOK FOR IN A SPINE FELLOWSHIP

If you are considering a fellowship in spine surgery, first outline what you want to accomplish. Then, when looking at different programs, determine the proportion of cases performed in deformity, pediatric, adult, and degenerative (cervical and/or lumbar) and trauma. If you are interested in learning about specific procedures, such as minimally invasive spinal surgery, intradural work, or tumor surgery, find out if the institution at which you may train performs an adequate volume of these procedures.

When interviewing, be sure to ask the fellows how they spend the majority of their time in the operating room: actively performing cases, or just observing? Also, do not overlook the importance of office hours. Time spent with the attending staff in the office or clinic setting is an important part of their fellowship experience. Here, the fellow learns about non-operative management, physical therapy protocols, and operative indications while improving upon physical examination and diagnostic skills. Fellowships vary greatly in this respect, so investigate this aspect of the experience carefully. Keep in mind that an important aspect of spine training is to learn the indications for different procedures, not simply learning how to perform them.

While many programs have a research requirement, the amount of actual work and the quality of projects varies considerably from program to program. Ask the fellows how much work is actually required and what kind of ancillary help is available to them. For those interested in academic careers, ask how many publications current and past fellows have produced.

The daily workload varies as well from program to program. In some programs, the fellows do not round at all. In some places, the fellows round with residents who help change dressings and take care of the daily patient responsibilities, and in other places, you are responsible for everything and the nurses call you directly with questions. Some places require fellows to take call. Ask how often call is, and whether the fellows round on the weekends. Some places require fellows to take general orthopedic call. This can be a valuable experience and can keep up your skills in general orthopedics, but can sometimes also detract from your specialty training.

Remember that there are more spots than applicants, so landing a spot shouldn't be too hard. While a small number of people do not match, there are usually a larger number of spots at programs that do not match, and some of them at programs that are usually considered more desirable. This means that you shouldn't rank programs that you do not really want to go to. Do not worry, if you are a good applicant, you will likely find a place even if you do not match.

APPLYING FOR A SPINE FELLOWSHIP

The Spine Surgery Fellowship Match (SFM) was established in 2008. The North American Spine Society (NASS) has sponsored the matching process. You can refer to www.sfmatch.org/fellowship/f_spn/index.htm for more information. The participating programs will not make any appointments until the Match has been completed. The function of the Matching Program is strictly limited to processing the Match. The decision to be listed or not rests solely with each individual program director. Registration begins in July (the beginning of the PGY-4). The registration form can be found at www.sfmatch.org/forms/registration/applicant/2010MatchRegFormFSPN.pdf.

After you register an on-line application, you will receive more information by e-mail. The CAS distributes applications to residency training programs. You need to fill out one universal application form, gather one copy of each of the appropriate documents, and mail your entire package to CAS. This application can be found at www.sfmatch.org/forms/cas/SPN_CASapplication.pdf.

You will need the following supporting documents:

1. Three letters of recommendations, one of which must be from the "residency program director"
2. Medical school dean's letter and references
3. College and medical school transcripts
4. United States Medical Licensing Examination (USMLE) scores (inclusion of Orthopaedic In-Training Exam [OITE] scores are optional)

The match system currently allows only 3 letters of recommendation, and the same letters are sent to every program, so make sure you make the most of this. Most people choose to get one letter from the chair of their orthopedic program, one from the chief of their spine service, and one from a well-known spine attending in their program whom they know well. It is helpful to identify these people as early as possible in residency and work with them in the OR, office hours, and research projects. Some people also mail additional letters of recommendation separately from the Match.

For your personal statement, be sure to have many people look this over for you, especially your spine department chair or others who have experience in the application process.

There is no deadline to apply as far as the Match is concerned, but most programs do have their own deadline. In general, most places wait until most of the applications have come in and then sit down and decide who they want to interview. This means that you do not have to apply the minute the match goes online, but do not wait too long either. You should review the Key Dates on the SFM Web site (www.sfmatch.org/fellowship/f_spn/getting_started/key_dates.htm) for more information. However, if you do end up applying late to a program, be sure to call that place to encourage them to take a look at your application.

The interviews take place sometime between January and March. Programs have 1, 2, or 3 interview dates. There will often be conflicts among available dates, and it can be tricky scheduling them. Sometimes programs interview during national meetings, so do not miss out on a good chance to interview and network. Good advice for fellowship interviews is the same as for residency interviews (see Chapter 6). This is your chance to talk with attendings and fellows about the program to find out if you will be happy spending a year there.

You should do a little research about the attending before you arrive, review the information about the program they sent you, and review your CV and personal statement. Know about the places you interview before you get there, because you want to maximize the brief amount of time you have during each interview and avoid asking questions whose answers are clearly stated in the program's informational packet. Expect to be asked about research you have conducted or case reports you have written, and prepare accordingly.

After the interview, be sure to write down the details. When it comes time to make your rank list, you'll be glad that you did. It is also a good idea to send a thank you email to the people who interviewed you. This should be done as soon as possible after the interview, certainly within a week or 2. You may also want to ask your chairperson or someone in your program to call the fellowship director and put in a good word for you. Letting a program know it is your first choice is a good idea, but never do this to more than one place.

Finally, maintain a rank-order list as you go through interviews. The rank list is submitted in March. The Match takes place in May and will be used to process all applicants who want to start their fellowship training in July of the following year. Keep in mind that fellowships do not always fill all of their positions, and some may become available after the Match. The vacancies are posted, and applicants who have not matched may begin negotiating directly with the program directors. The vacancies are listed at www.sfmatch.org/vacancies/f_spine.htm.

MUSCULOSKELETAL ONCOLOGY FELLOWSHIP

A match has recently been organized for musculoskeletal oncology fellowships in conjunction with the adult reconstructive hip and knee fellowship. The match is administered by the SF Match (www.sfmatch.org) and sponsored by the American Association of Hip and Knee Surgeons (AAHKS), the Hip Society (HS), the Knee Society (KS), and the Musculoskeletal Tumor Society (MSTS). Go to www.aahks.org for more information regarding the match, including deadlines and a universal application.

The MSTS keeps a master list of fellowships updated on their Web site (http://msts.org). Individual programs may require you to submit a copy of the universal application along with letters of recommendation and your CV. As with the reconstructive fellowship, this will allow you to interview at multiple programs, and it "levels the playing field," optimizing your chances at training at the fellowship of your choice.

Job Search: What to Look for in a Potential Position

Looking for a job can be a daunting task, engendering anxiety even in the calmest of individuals. Academic, private practice (large group versus small group), multispecialty group, solo private practice, and health maintenance organization (HMO) groups—each has its own set of pros and cons. Ultimately, your job selection may have little to do with anything other than location and spouse preference. Also, it is likely that your first job will not be your last.

The first step while you are in your fellowship or last year of general training is to be honest with yourself and ask yourself some very basic questions. Then you can break down the pros and cons of each selection and how it fits into your lifestyle.

DO YOU WANT TO SPECIALIZE IN A SPECIFIC SUBSPECIALTY AT YOUR JOB?

The answer to this question is not always straightforward. Jobs allowing you to do only your specific subspecialty training are rare unless they are academic. Some private practices may be structured to allow you to focus entirely on your subspecialty training, but these are rare. More than likely, you will be able to have a focus in your practice but also need to do general orthopedics.

WHAT PRACTICE TYPE ARE YOU LOOKING FOR?

Available options include academic, private practice, HMO, and Veterans Affairs (VA)/military. Private practice options break down further into small groups, orthopedic surgeon-only groups, and multispecialty groups. Academic practices also have a strict salary agreement versus incentive-based agreements.

PRACTICE LOCATION AND SPOUSE/FAMILY DESIRE

Are you interested in working in a rural area, major city, suburb, beach, or mountain area? Do not underestimate your spouse's desires!

Laith M. Jazrawi, MD

L. M. Jazrawi, K. A. Egol, & J. D. Zuckerman.
Orthopedic Residency & Fellowship: A Guide to Success (pp. 127-130)
© 2010 Taylor & Francis Group.

Chapter 18

As you filter through these issues, it is important to make your pro/con list. At the 2009 American Academy of Orthopaedic Surgeons (AAOS) annual meeting, Allan Mishra, in his Instructional Course, put together a nice pro/con list of available practice options, which is listed in Table 18-1.[1]

Table 18-1

PRACTICE SELECTION MATRIX

PRACTICE TYPE	PROS	CONS
Academic Practice	• Teaching of residents • Research potential • Coverage of patients by residents • Ability to pursue a subspecialty • Collaboration with other specialists	• Time commitment without reimbursement for teaching • Pressure to publish • Grant applications • Still have need to produce clinically • Committee or university responsibilities
Private Practice—Large Group (6-25+ surgeons)	• Better negotiating with managed care • More availability for mentor relationships • Income may be higher due to ancillary service income • Less call coverage but more intense	• Too many surgeons may create difficult practice governance • May only be able to pursue narrow specialty • Internal referrals may be tilted toward older partners
Private Practice—Small Group (2-5 surgeons)	• Right combination of expertise in group may be ideal • Easier to make practice decisions • Compensation typically better than multispecialty practice • Accountability of staff to surgeons	• Less negotiating power with managed care • Personality conflicts may arise • Call coverage more often • Internal competition for patients may result
Private Practice—Solo	• Ability to make all practice decisions	• Need to cover all call or arrange coverage • Difficult managed care contracting • Need to arrange all of the business aspects of practice
Multispecialty Group	• Built-in referral base • Ability to seek consults from all other medical specialties as needed	• Less compensation • Likely need to be a general orthopedist • Practice governance usually dominated by primary care physicians
Closed HMO	• Good starting salaries • Busy practice immediately • Reasonable call schedules • Excellent benefits and pension	• Fixed working hours • Practiced controlled by HMO • No outside patients • No equity opportunity • Limited ability to benefit from ancillary services
Institutional Military/VA	• Excellent electronic medical record • Serving veterans • Immediately busy case load • Potential for travel	• Potential for deployment to war zone • Lower salaries • Highly bureaucratic • Very little control over cases or clinics

Reproduced with permission from Mishra A, Urquhart AG, Anders T. Selecting and starting an orthopaedic surgery practice. In: Duwelius PJ, Azar FM, eds. *Instructional Course Lectures 57.* Rosemont, IL: American Academy of Orthopaedic Surgeons; 2008:729-736.

Once you have gone through your checklist, certain factors will hold more weight with you depending on your background. Remember that no decision needs to be final, and changing jobs is okay. You need to make certain that your contract (see Chapter 19) is written to protect you in case this happens. Good luck!

REFERENCE

1. Mishra A, Davis S, Jorgensen A, LaRoque E. Key issues in starting your orthopaedic practice. *Instr Course Lect*. 2009 AAOS Annual Meeting.

REVIEWING PHYSICIAN EMPLOYMENT CONTRACTS

After many years of representing physicians who are signing their first employment contract (for purposes of this article, I will refer to those physicians as "junior physicians"), I am still amazed by how many physicians will sign the contract without consulting with a lawyer or even understanding some of the basic terms that are contained in the contract. It is important to understand that, in most cases, your future employer has hired an attorney to draft the contract, and that lawyer is not looking out for your interests but for the interest of the group you are joining.

I am not suggesting that all contracts are bad or that most medical practices are trying to harm those junior physicians they hire, but, as discussed next, even a standard contract can have significant financial ramifications on you during the term of the contract (eg, Will you be on call every weekend in the event you decide to leave? Or, will you have to pay thousands of dollars if you leave to purchase a "malpractice tail endorsement?") and on your ability to practice in the future (eg, Are you subject to a large restrictive covenant?).

If a practice tells you that it will look negatively on your chances of joining the group if you attempt to request changes or if you consult with a lawyer, then you have your first clue on whether this group is right for you. A group may tell you the contract is non-negotiable, but this does not mean you should not understand the contract and be able to ask questions. A group that wants junior physicians to be robots and just sign what is put in front of them may not be an ideal situation. At the same time, it is important to have an advisor who can guide you in identifying the crucial issues to raise with the employer and the less important ones that you will "just see how things turn out." In my years of representing medical practices (which I do in addition to representing junior physicians), there have been instances where junior physicians are overly aggressive or "nitpicky," and this has caused the employer to looks less favorably on the applicant. Bottom line: you need to figure out which battles are worth fighting over in the contract.

Below is an overview of certain major provisions that should be the subject of your attention. We have also provided some suggestions to help you avoid making common mistakes in negotiating an initial employment contract.

Andrew E. Blustein, Esq

L. M. Jazrawi, K. A. Egol, & J. D. Zuckerman.
Orthopedic Residency & Fellowship: A Guide to Success (pp. 131-134)
© 2010 Taylor & Francis Group.

RESPONSIBILITIES/ON CALL

A contract should clearly delineate the responsibilities of the junior physician to the practice. Some contracts will specify the number of hours that are expected, although this is becoming less common. Many contracts will simply state that the job is a full-time commitment and may contain a restriction on outside activities. The junior physician needs to consider whether he or she intends to have other commitments and, if so, negotiate a "carve-out."

One of the most controversial issues is the physician's on-call obligations. Some contracts will include a specific on-call schedule or a statement indicating that "on call" will be divided equally. Generally, either approach is acceptable. If the on-call responsibilities in the contract are vague, the junior physician's attorney should address the issue. Many practices will, however, take the position that call is not equal. For example, senior physicians may take no call or reduced call. This is a factor that the junior physician needs to take into account when deciding which practice to join.

TERMINATION EVENTS

Physician agreements often include provisions permitting the practice to terminate the junior physician without cause after the practice provides notice of termination. Some contracts lengthen or eliminate the right to terminate without cause after several years have passed. While the junior physician's attorney may be able to negotiate for more notice time, the effect of a without-cause termination can still be considerable: the junior physician may suddenly have to look for a new job. As explained in detail below, this situation could become more difficult if the recent junior is subject to a *restrictive covenant*. The junior physician needs to appreciate this insecurity, although it is unlikely to be removed from most contracts.

Most contracts also contain provisions that permit the practice to terminate the junior physician for specific "for-cause" events. This termination is usually triggered on much shorter notice than without-cause termination. A typical contract can devote up to a page or more describing many "for-cause" events. Some termination events are obvious, such as a breach of stated obligations or loss of a medical license. Other events may involve failure to obtain privileges in certain hospitals, which is why it is important for the junior physician to obtain these privileges *before* the start date of the contract if possible. Still other events may be highly subjective and provide the practice with the right to terminate employment for other reasons deemed important. The attorney for the junior physician should attempt to provide the employee with the ability to solve these issues before termination becomes effective and also to narrow the scope of these provisions.

SALARY/COMPENSATION

The question we are asked most frequently by junior physicians is whether we believe the salary in their contract is reasonable. This is a difficult question to answer for several reasons. First, while junior physicians tend to be familiar with what they perceive as the "going rate," the rate varies depending on location (eg, rural versus major metropolitan area) and medical specialty. Second, and most important, a contract may offer a lower salary but actually be a better opportunity. For example, a practice may offer a lower salary, but the contract may contain a shorter period to partnership with a lower buy-in price for the ownership interest. The cliché that "all that glitters is not gold" is very true in the context of selecting the right contract.

Incentive compensation is another area of concern for graduating physicians. There are many different formulas for incentive compensation, but the most typical is to provide the graduating physician with a percentage of collections (eg, 15%) above a specified dollar threshold (eg, $400,000). Many junior physicians become too focused on the dollar amounts (eg, 20% instead of 15%), but the junior physician is rarely in a position to determine if the practice has selected a realistic goal. The answer to this question will often arrive at the end of the first year, and that is why we suggest that a junior physician monitor whether this goal is likely to be obtained after 6 to 8 months into the contract year.

OPPORTUNITY FOR PARTNERSHIP

Many employment contracts will not promise the junior physician that he or she will be made an owner of the practice. In fact, many contracts may end after 1 or 2 years. Other contracts may provide a timetable for partnership, but state that this partnership is available "only if offered by the practice." In both of these cases, the junior physician has no guarantee of partnership. For this reason, the graduating physician has to understand that he or she generally cannot be assured a future with the practice after the end of the contract. An attorney representing the junior physician can attempt to negotiate provisions to remove some of the uncertainty. Also, the attorney should attempt to add a provision about the amount of the "buy-in" you may pay if you are offered partnership. The trend in many groups, however, is not to provide significant detail toward what the future partnership may look like.

MALPRACTICE INSURANCE

Many states have 2 types of malpractice insurance. The more beneficial is *occurrence insurance*, which will protect the physician with coverage whenever the action is brought, so long as the coverage was in place when any alleged malpractice occurred, even if it is brought after the contract is terminated or expires. The second type is *claims-made insurance*, which will only provide coverage if the policy with the same insurer is in effect 1) when the malpractice was committed and 2) when the actual action is commenced. While claims-made insurance is cheaper, the junior physician can be left without coverage if he or she leaves the practice and does not maintain the same insurance policy. For this reason, the attorney for the junior physician will want the practice to purchase an occurrence policy, but this is often not offered.

The good news is that claims-made insurance can often be converted into occurrence insurance by the purchase of something called a *tail endorsement*. The bad news is that a tail endorsement can cost thousands of dollars. Therefore, one of the most crucial issues in an employment contract that includes claims-made insurance coverage will be whether the junior physician or the practice bears the cost for the tail endorsement. An experienced health care attorney will be able to suggest some compromise positions so that the payments for the tail may be shared with the practice. Also, insurance policies vary among insurance companies and states, so these general rules may need to be changed.

RESTRICTIVE COVENANT

A restrictive covenant is a contract provision stating that an employee cannot work for a given amount of time after the contract terminates or expires (eg, 2 years) within a given restrictive zone (eg, 4 miles from each of the offices of the practice). The provision may also require the physician to resign hospital privileges. Over the years, many physicians have said they believe that these provisions are unenforceable; however, these beliefs are often incorrect. While the laws of the state in which the practice is located typically govern these provisions, most states will enforce a *reasonably* drafted restrictive covenant. What is considered "reasonable" is something that should be discussed with an attorney, but it is important for the junior physician to understand the size of the restricted area and the potential effect of the covenant. In the vast majority of contracts, a junior physician should expect to agree to a restrictive covenant of some kind and should consider these provisions in evaluating different contracts.

BENEFITS

A thorough discussion of the benefits that a junior physician often receives is beyond the scope of this article. However, health insurance is often provided by the practice to the junior physician, although family coverage is not always given. Disability insurance is another important benefit; but it is important to recognize that an employee may be taxed on any disability payments he or she receives under a policy that was provided as a benefit by and at the expense of the practice. For this reason, the junior physician may want to purchase a supplemental policy or consider some other alternative (eg, if possible, opt out of the practice's policy and receive a higher salary). Many other benefits, such as vacation, vary greatly between different contracts. It is important for the graduating physician to understand his or her benefits, but most practices will want to retain their ability to alter benefits during the contract term.

CONCLUSION

The junior physician needs to understand his or her employment contract before it is executed. Most contracts contain clauses that state that any promises not included in the contract are unenforceable. For this reason, if you find that an important understanding is not part of the contract, it needs to be included in the contract as part of the negotiation process. Unfortunately, a junior physician who signs a contract on "trust" may find out that if there is an acrimonious parting of the ways with the practice, the contract can be used to attack the junior physician or deprive him or her of benefits that were expected. A clearly drafted and balanced contract can increase the chances that the event can be peaceful and non-confrontational if the junior physician separates from the practice.

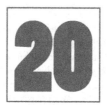

THE BOARDS

Patients and society in general expect the highest commitment to excellence when it comes to their health care. Specialty board certification is a process that demonstrates an individual practitioner's commitment to excellence. In addition, many insurance panels as well as hospitals require board certification for their doctors in order to be credentialed. Board certification is not mandatory and thereby differs from state licensure. This specific credential, however, is the "gold standard" when it comes to the practice of orthopedic surgery in the United States. The American Board of Orthopaedic Surgeons (ABOS) is a separate organization from the American Academy of Orthopaedic Surgeons (AAOS) and is charged with certifying that orthopedic surgeons have met certain quality standards in training, education, and practice. The ABOS certifying examination has 2 sections—a written (Part I) and oral examination (Part II). The ABOS is designed to evaluate the initial and continuing qualifications and knowledge of orthopedic surgeons. The examination is statistically valid only as a pass/fail test. The test is not designed to compare percentile scores among residents or throughout different years. To remain accredited, orthopedic residency programs must have a pass rate of at least 75% on the ABOS Part I examination for residents taking the test for the first time. In order to sit for the board examinations, a candidate must be a graduate of an accredited 4-year medical school, have successfully completed a minimum 5-year accredited residency program in the United States or Canada (with appropriate documentation), and the final 24 months of training must have been obtained from a single training program. In addition, all applicants must have an unrestricted license or a government work permit where a license is not required.

WRITTEN EXAMINATION
Kenneth A. Egol, MD

Orthopedic surgeons who have completed an accredited residency, as attested by the program director to the ABOS credentials committee, may apply and be admitted to take the written examination. This examination, which is a timed, secure, paper and pencil exam, consists of approximately 320 multiple choice questions covering all of orthopedics. It is currently given at the Hyatt hotel in Chicago on a single day in July. It involves 7 hours of testing divided into 2 sessions. The content outline for the most recent examination is available at www.abos.org. In the future, it will be given on the computer at select test centers across the country.

L. M. Jazrawi, K. A. Egol, & J. D. Zuckerman.
Orthopedic Residency & Fellowship: A Guide to Success (pp. 135-144)
© 2010 Taylor & Francis Group.

The questions are produced through the work of more than 70 volunteer practicing orthopedic surgeons, with the help and professional guidance of the National Board of Medical Examiners (NBME). Each question submitted is required to be supported by at least 2 peer-reviewed references and is subject to review by at least 3 different groups of surgeons before appearing on a test: the Question Writing Task Force (QWTF), the Field Test Task Force (FTTF), and the written exam committee of the ABOS. Extensive statistics are kept by the NBME on the performance of each question, and poorly performing questions (too hard, too easy, non-discriminating) are discarded. The passing score is set each year by the written exam committee based on an item-by-item analysis and the work of yet another group of volunteer orthopedic surgeons, the standard setting task force. The overall pass rate in recent years has varied from 79% to 88%. The pass rate for US/Canadian medical school graduates taking the test for the first time is substantially higher. More information about the written exam is available at www.abos.org.

After passing Part I, candidates have a period of 5 years to apply for and pass the Part II oral examination. If they do not, they must re-take Part I to be admitted to the oral exam. It is each candidate's responsibility to know deadlines and make a correct, complete application if he or she wishes to be board certified. In order to be admitted to the oral examination, a candidate must have a full and unrestricted medical license and have been in practice for at least 22 months, of which at least 12 are in a single location. The Board will obtain peer review of the candidate from certified orthopedic surgeons who are familiar with his or her work and get evaluations from the hospital chief of staff, chief of orthopedics, surgery, anesthesia, and nursing staff in the operating room and orthopedic wards. This information is reviewed by the credentials committee of the ABOS, who will decide which applicants are admitted to sit for the Part II examination.

Multiple studies have included ABOS examination performance as an outcome measure for orthopedic resident success because the exam provides a nationwide objective means for evaluating residents. Dirschl and colleagues used the ABOS Part I percentile score as a means to measure resident success.[1] The study found that none of the predictors studied correlated with ABOS performance. Dirschl et al also found that there was little internal correlation between ABOS Part I scores and overall resident performance based on faculty evaluations. The study concluded that ABOS scores may not be good outcome measures of resident performance.[1] Thordarson and colleagues also found that ABOS scores do not correlate with faculty performance evaluations or any of the predictive factors studied.[2] Turner and colleagues did report that the Quantitative Composite Scoring System used to predict future applicant success significantly predicted ABOS written and oral examination pass/fail status.[3] Analysis of our residency program's experience with trying to identify which residents pass the Part I exam did not find any significant relationship between any predictors studied and ABOS examination results. The Orthopaedic In-Training Exam (OITE) scores did not correlate with passing the ABOS Part I exam, likely because of the extremely high rate of passage in this program (97%).

In 2007, Thordarson et al ranked 46 former residents of 4 consecutive residency classes at the author's home institution from best qualified to least qualified upon acceptance into the program.[2] The initial rank list was based on 9 criteria that the 4 faculty members on the resident selection committee felt were important. Upon resident completion of the training program, the same 4 faculty members ranked the residents again based on overall residency performance and compared the results of the 2 lists. The rankings of the residents were also compared to their respective United States Medical Licensing Examination (USMLE) Step 1 scores, ABOS Part I scores, fourth-year OITE scores, and "Best Doctor" award. Statistical analysis showed that resident OITE and ABOS scores were strongly correlated. However, fair to poor correlations were found between initial rank and final rank list order. USMLE Step 1 scores showed poor to fair correlation with ABOS and OITE scores. Faculty members were in relative agreement in regard to applicant selection criteria, but disagreed on the final rankings of residents.

Preparation for an exam of this type must begin well in advance of the end of the fifth post-graduate year (PGY-5). The essential foundations needed to pass the board examination begin in the PGY-1 year and continue throughout residency. While no one can learn the breadth of material needed to pass this exam in 1 week, many graduating residents opt for a boards review course. These courses are designed to provide an intense overview of all facets of orthopedic surgery and clinical and basic science. They are usually given over a 3- to 5-day period with syllabi provided.

REVIEW COURSES

AAOS Board Preparation and Review Course
6300 North River Road
Rosemont, IL 60018-4262
Phone: (800) 626-6726
www.aaos.org/education/education.asp

Johns Hopkins Orthopaedic Review
Johns Hopkins Outpatient Center
601 North Caroline Street, #5240
Baltimore, MD 21287
Phone: (410) 955-3870
Fax: (410) 955-1719
www.hopkinsortho.org/courses.html

Maine Orthopaedic Review
Maine Orthopaedic Course
PO Box 156
Gorham, ME 04038
Phone: (800) 792-0003
www.maineorthopaedic.com

Miller Orthopaedic Review Course
Miller Orthopaedic Research & Education
1586 Lily Lake Drive
Colorado Springs, CO 80921
Phone: (866) 615-6376 or (719) 495-8249
Fax: (866) 847-4089 or (719) 574-0006
www.millerreview.org

REFERENCES

1. Dirschl DR, Campion ER, Gilliam K. Resident selection and predictors of performance: can we be evidence based? *Clin Orthop*. 2006;449:44-49.
2. Thordarson DB, Ebramzadeh E, Sangiorgio SN, Schnall SB, Patzakis MJ. Resident selection: how are we doing and why? *Clin Orthop*. 2007;459:255-259.
3. Turner NS, Shaughnessy WJ, Berg EJ, Larson DR, Hanssen AD. A quantitative composite scoring tool for orthopaedic residency screening and selection. *Clin Orthop*. 2006;449:50-55.

ORAL EXAMINATION

Laith M. Jazrawi, MD

After completing your residency training and finishing and hopefully passing Part I of the ABOS examination, most of you will move to fellowship and delay thinking about ABOS Part II. The ABOS was founded in 1934 to serve the public interest by examining orthopedic surgeons and certifying that they have met set standards of education, practice, and training. Board certification continues to be a separate and distinct process from your state licensing exam and is a voluntary process. However, board certification is the gold standard for medical specialization in the United States and often is a required credential for hospital privileges, AAOS membership, medical insurance plan participation, and other credentialing matters.

ABOS certification is received after passing Part II of the Board examination, which is an oral test. Educational criteria required for board certification include 1) graduating from an accredited 4-year medical school and 2) successfully completing a minimum 5-year accredited orthopedic residency program in the United States or Canada with the final 2 years of training obtained in a single program. Applicants for Part II of the Boards must have a full and unrestricted license to practice medicine and have been in practice for at least 22 months, of which at least 12 are in a single location. The Board will obtain peer review of the candidate from certified orthopedic surgeons who are familiar with his or her work and get evaluations from the hospital chief of staff; chief of orthopedics, surgery, and anesthesia; and nursing staff in the operating room and orthopedic wards. This information is reviewed by the credentials committee of the ABOS, who will decide which applicants are admitted to sit for the Part II examination. Once you have passed the written examination (Part I), you are deemed "board eligible" until successful completion of Part II. The limit of board eligibility is 5 years. If Part II is not passed within 5 years of passing Part I, you must re-take and pass Part I again before applying for Part II.

The oral examination is based on all cases collected during a 6-month period. The cases are submitted electronically through a program called "Scribe." Twelve cases are selected. The candidate can choose 10 of those 12 to present during the oral examination. The exam is administered yearly in July at the Palmer House Hotel in Chicago. You will need to bring 3 copies of all pertinent medical records and 1 copy of imaging studies for each of the 10 cases. There are three 35-minute examination sessions conducted by 2 examiners each. The examiners independently grade each case presentation on 6 skills: data gathering and interpretation, diagnosis, treatment plan, technical skill, outcomes, and applied knowledge. In addition, the case list is evaluated on surgical indications, handling of complications, ethics, and professionalism. While a majority of the applicants are fellowship trained, most applicants test in the general orthopedic panel. Subspecialty panels include trauma, spine, hand, pediatrics, foot and ankle, and sports. Applications and the case list collection program are available April 1 of each year and are due in October. Candidates who pass the examination are notified in the fall. After passing Part II, a surgeon receives a certificate and becomes a "diplomate" of the ABOS for 10 years.

There are several issues that remain paramount during the time leading up to the oral exam. First is the 6-month collection period. While this can be a source of great consternation, the goal is to continue to practice orthopedics in a fundamentally clinically sound way based on standard of care practices established during your residency and fellowship training and supported in the literature. In other words, practice orthopedics like you should always be practicing it. To exhaust nonsurgical management on a patient who clearly needs surgical intervention based on current standard of care practices because you want to be ultra-conservative and show your reviewers that you are not quick to cut is counterproductive to good patient care. There will be cases that clearly are more controversial and may be better dealt with by your partner or associate or referred out if you feel uncomfortable managing it. However, even the most challenging of cases and even the worst complications, if dealt with in the appropriate manner and recognized in a timely manner, will not result in failure. The reviewers will not fail you simply because of poor outcome or complications. Poor ethical decisions and inappropriate management of a complication is more a cause for concern. Remember, the reviewers are there to make decisions based on data gathering and interpretation, diagnosis, treatment plan, technical skill, outcomes, and applied knowledge. In surgical indications (handling of complications and ethics and professionalism), the reviewers are more likely to criticize incomplete information and inadequate documentation as reasons for failure. During the 6-month collection, it is critically important to clearly document in all office notes and hospital notes your reasoning behind pursuing your method of treatment and a clear, logical approach to dealing with the problem. The motto "if you think it, write it down" is important for you because it provides detailed support to your plan of care and also allows the hospital to bill the appropriate level of care and get the appropriate reimbursement if everything is clearly documented. In addition, make copies of all of your radiologic studies, arthroscopic photos, and surgery cases during your collections period. This will save you time later on gathering x-rays and magnetic resonance imaging (MRI).

For those of you who are in the academic world or cover a local non-private hospital, make certain you follow up on the care of these patients even though the residents are caring for them. Ultimately, any complications need to be mentioned and included and appropriate follow-up detailed. It is normal to be anxious about the oral examination. However, remember that you have successfully completed medical school, residency, your USMLE exams, and Part I of the ABOS. Treat it like a conference during your orthopedic residency when you were pumped with questions about patient management. Last, as a final piece of comfort, the pass rate averages 90%. Good luck!

MAINTENANCE OF CERTIFICATION

Joseph D. Zuckerman, MD

After successfully completing ABOS Part I (written) and Part II (oral) examinations, you become a diplomate of the ABOS, or "board certified." Prior to 1986, board certification was a lifetime certificate, and recertification was not required. However, all orthopedic surgeons certified in 1986 and later receive 10-year certificates. Each diplomate of the ABOS with a time-limited certificate is required to recertify within 10 years. Successful completion of a recertification exam provided an additional 10-year certificate. The concept of time-limited certificates and recertification reflects the goals of "lifelong learning." As physicians, to fulfill our contract with society and maintain the public trust, we should be involved in continued learning and improvement so that we can provide the best possible care for our patients. The recertification process is now referred to as *maintenance of certification* or MOC. MOC is the process through which diplomates of the ABOS maintain their "board certification" in orthopedic surgery.

MOC developed in response to external regulatory forces as well as public demand. After the American Board of Medical Specialties (ABMS) defined the general competencies of a competent physician (medical knowledge, patient care, interpersonal and communication skills, professionalism, practice-based learning and improvement, and systems-based practice), each member board was required to develop methods to systematically assess these competencies on a periodic basis as part of the MOC process. Whereas recertification initially only required an examination every 10 years, the MOC process is now designed to assess the general competencies in a systematic way. Currently, the ABOS defines 4 components of MOC as follows:

1. Evidence of professional standing
2. Evidence of lifelong learning and self-assessment
3. Evidence of cognitive expertise
4. Evidence of performance and practice

The ABOS is currently in transition as it fully integrates the 4-component MOC process. The full MOC process is in place for those who received board certification in 2010 or whose board certification expires in 2010. There are specific requirements that must be fulfilled during the 10-year process (Figure 20-1). However, in order to better understand the process, let's discuss the components of MOC.

1. *Evidence of professional standing*: This will require that each diplomate maintain a full and unrestricted license to practice medicine in the United States or Canada.

2. *Evidence of lifelong learning and self-assessment*: This will be addressed through ongoing 3-year cycles of 120 credits of Category I orthopedic or relevant continuing medical education (CME) that will include a minimum of 20 CME credits of self-assessment examinations (SAE). It is important that these self-assessment examinations be "scored and recorded." This can best be accomplished by using the self-assessment exams developed by AAOS. However, when obtaining these exams, it is important to elect the "scored and recorded" option. The ABOS requirement is for completion and scoring of self-assessment examinations; however, the SAEs do not have a passing or a failing grade. The goal is to use the SAE scoring to help direct your study plan as part of your personal quality improvement program. The only documentation that you have to provide the ABOS is that you have completed and returned for scoring the required number of SAE credits.

   Fulfilling the requirements of lifelong learning and assessment requires an accurate documentation of Category I CME credits. It will be important for each diplomate to keep track of all CME credits earned. This process can be facilitated by the AAOS. For details, you should contact the AAOS to enroll in the MOC documentation process. It is also important to note that documentation of CME credits must be reported directly to the ABOS. Detailed instructions are available on the ABOS Web site.

3. *Evidence of cognitive expertise*: This occurs through a secure examination as has been used for recertification since the early 1990s. This option can include either a written examination or an oral examination. The specific details about these options will be discussed later in this chapter.

MOC Process with Computer or Oral Examination Pathway

	Year 1	Year 2	Year 3	Year 4	Year 5	Year 6	Year 7	Year 8	Year 9	Year 10
Lifelong Learning and Self-Assessment	Total of 120 Category I CME Credits • Topics may include orthopaedics, ethics, professionalism, cultural competence • Minimum of 20 credits from Scored and Recorded Self-Assessment Examination(s)			Total of 120 Category I CME Credits • Topics may include orthopaedics, ethics, professionalism, cultural competence • Minimum of 20 credits from Scored and Recorded Self-Assessment Examination(s)			Additional CME as necessary for state licensure requirements			
Cognitive Expertise							File Application with ABOS	Secure Computer Examination or Oral Examination Pathway from ABOS		
Professional Standing							Credentialing and Peer Review			
Performance in Practice						Case List (Computer Exam Path)	Case List (Oral Exam Path)			

Figure 20-1. This 10-year schedule depicts the MOC process for diplomates. Contact the ABOS for specific information about your year of certification and related MOC requirements and deadlines. Reprinted with permission. American Academy of Orthopaedic Surgeons. Data source: The American Board of Orthopaedic Surgery.

4. *Evaluation of performance and practice*: This will include a stringent peer-review process and will use performance indicators including sign-your-site, preoperative antibiotics, informed consent, and postoperative anticoagulation. The credentials committee of the ABOS plans to expand its peer-review process to include patient questionnaires that address doctor-patient communication skills as well as patient satisfaction. These questionnaires are currently being developed by the ABMS. The quality improvement focus of the fourth component of the MOC will also begin to evaluate diplomates' participation in programs and practices that deliver better and safer patient care.

OPTIONS FOR COMPLETION OF THE "SECURE EXAMINATION" REQUIREMENT

At present (2010), the ABOS offers 6 options to fulfill the secure examination requirement. Five options involve a written examination, and the sixth option is an oral examination. The written examination options are all practice profile/specialty oriented, multiple choice, computer-based examinations. Five specific computer-based exams are offered including the following:

1. General orthopedic surgery
2. Adult reconstructive surgery
3. Spine surgery
4. Orthopedic sports medicine
5. Hand surgery—This examination is available only to those individuals who hold a subspecialty certificate in surgery of the hand.

All of the specialty computer-based examinations (options 2 through 5) include questions on "core orthopedic knowledge" including topics related to ethics and patient communication. These questions comprise 40% of each examination. The content of the core orthopedic knowledge questions are listed in Table 20-1.[1]

The sixth option is a practice-based oral examination. This is available for orthopedic surgeons who continue to engage in the operative care of patients. This option requires submission of case lists from which a specific group of cases are selected for presentation to oral examiners. This examination generally takes place in July in Chicago. If this recertification option is selected, the ABOS will also consider it as fulfilling the requirements for the fourth component of MOC—evaluation of performance and practice.

The practice profile computer-based written examinations are generally available during 2 months each year—March and April—at various testing sites across the country. The examination for those individuals with a certificate of added qualifications in surgery of the hand is available during a 4-week period in the fall. Additional details concerning these examinations are available at the ABOS Web site (www.abos.org).

Those of you reading this book are still a number of years from achieving initial board certification in orthopedic surgery. Keep in mind that the MOC process begins after you achieve board certification. It is at that point that the 10-year cycle begins. It is quite possible that the guidelines presented in this chapter will change by that time. Therefore, it is important that you obtain the most up-to-date information from the ABOS at the time you become board certified.

Table 20-1

COMPONENTS BY TOPIC OF THE "CORE ORTHOPEDIC KNOWLEDGE" QUESTIONS ON THE COMPUTER-BASED SPECIALTY RECERTIFICATION EXAMINATIONS

1) GENERAL ITEMS	15-30%
a. Legal/ethical	1-3%
b. Basic science principles	2-4%
c. Multiple trauma (non-orthopedic), (ie, traumatic brain injury, etc)	10-15%
d. Postoperative complications	1-3%
e. Rheumatologic conditions	0-1%
f. Miscellaneous (child abuse, etc)	2-4%
2) UPPER EXTREMITY	**15-30%**
a. Fractures of shoulder girdle	0-2%
b. Shoulder instabilities, arthritis, osteonecrosis	5-7%
c. Elbow fractures and arthritis	3-5%
d. Radius and ulna fractures, infection, etc	4-6%
e. Wrist injury, nerve compression	1-3%
f. Hand fractures, tendon injuries	5%
3) LOWER EXTREMITY	**35-54%**
a. Pelvis and acetabular fracture	3-5%
b. Hip dislocation/fractures, arthritis, pediatric problems	8-10%
c. Femur fracture	4%
d. Knee joint dislocation, fracture, osteonecrosis, cartilage disorders, patellofemoral problems	10-15%
e. Tibia/fibula injuries	3-5%
f. Ankle	3-5%
g. Foot arthritis, nerve compression, inflammatory condition, congenital and developmental disorders	4-6%
4) SPINE	**2%**
a. Fractures, arthritis, stenosis, disc disease	
5) TUMOR AND TUMOR-LIKE CONDITIONS	**3-5%**

Reproduced with permission from the American Board of Orthopaedic Surgery. Content of "Core Orthopaedic Knowledge" for all ABOS computer recertification examination pathways. Available at: https://www.abos.org/documents/Core_Recert_Questions_Content.pdf. Accessed December 16, 2009.

RESULTS OF RECERTIFICATION EXAMS

In general, the results of recertification examinations show a higher pass rate than the initial written and oral certification exams. As of this writing, the most recent information provided by the ABOS is for the 2008 exams. In 2008, a total of 957 orthopedic surgeons completed recertification exams of any type, and 922 (96%) passed.[2] There were 893 orthopedic surgeons who took 1 of the 5 written examinations, and 864 (97%) passed.[2] The passing rate for each individual written examination ranged from 96% to 99% as follows[2]:

- ✓ General Recertification Examination   96%
- ✓ Adult Reconstruction Recertification Examination   99%
- ✓ Sports Medicine Recertification Examination   98%
- ✓ Spine Recertification Examination   97%
- ✓ Hand Recertification Examination   96%

In 2008, 64 orthopedic surgeons used a practice-based oral recertification pathway. Of these, 58 passed for a passing rate of 90%.[2] These results show a higher pass rate for the written examinations compared with the oral examinations. This has been the pattern of results reported each year and may be a factor in deciding which recertification pathway you select. When the time comes for you to decide which recertification pathway to use, you should visit the ABOS Web site for the most recent data concerning the results of the recertification examinations.

MOC is an important part of the practice of orthopedic surgery. It indicates each orthopedic surgeon's commitment to lifelong learning in the care of our patients. After you successfully complete your certification exams, you will begin the 10-year MOC process. There will be requirements to be completed during these 10 years, and it will be important for you to be knowledgeable about not only the requirements but also the dates for completion. This information can be most easily obtained from the ABOS Web site. Preparing and completing the MOC process can be facilitated by coordinating your efforts with the AAOS.

REFERENCES

1. American Board of Orthopaedic Surgery. Content of "Core Orthopedic Knowledge" for all ABOS computer recertification examination pathways. Available at: https://www.abos.org/documents/Core_Recert_Questions_Content.pdf. Accessed December 16, 2009.
2. American Board of Orthopaedic Surgery. Exam statistics. Available at: https://www.abos.org/ModDefault.aspx?module=Diplomates&section=RecertExamStat. Accessed December 16, 2009.

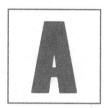

Accredited US Orthopedic Surgery Residency Programs

Alabama

University of Alabama Medical Center Program
Program Director: Steven M. Theiss, MD
University of Alabama Hospital
510 20th Street South
Faculty Office Tower #940
Birmingham, AL 35294
Tel: (205) 930-8494
Residency Coordinator: Vicki Allen
vicki.allen@ortho.uab.edu
PGY-1 Positions: 6
Required Research Year? No
Electives? No
http://medicine.uab.edu

University of South Alabama Program
Program Director: Frederick N. Meyer
University of South Alabama Hospitals
3421 Medical Park Drive
Department of Orthopaedic Surgery
2 Medical Park
Mobile, AL 36693
Tel: (251) 665-8250
Residency Coordinator: Gail M. Driver
gdriver@usamail.usouthal.edu
PGY-1 Positions: 2
Required Research Year? No
Electives? No
http://www.southalabama.edu

Arizona

Banner Good Samaritan Medical Center Program
Program Director: Alex C. McLaren, MD
Orthopedic Residency
1300 N 12 Street, Suite 620
Phoenix, AZ 85006
Tel: (602) 239-3671
Residency Coordinator: Laurel E. Kechanin
Orthopedic.residency@bannerhealth.com
PGY-1 Positions: 4
Required Research Year? No
Electives? No
http://www.bannerhealth.com

University of Arizona Program
Program Director: John T. Ruth, MD
Arizona Health Science Center
Department of Orthopaedic Surgery
PO Box 245064
Tucson, AZ 85724-5064
Tel: (520) 626-9245
Residency Coordinator: Susan J. Brandes
brandess@email.arizona.edu
PGY-1 Positions: 3
Required Research Year? No
Electives? No
http://www.bones.arizona.edu

Arkansas

University of Arkansas for Medical Sciences Program
Program Director: R. Dale Blasier, MD, MBA
University of Arkansas for Medical Sciences
4301 W. Markham Street, Slot 531
Little Rock, AR 72205
Tel: (501) 686-5251
Residency Coordinator: Darlene M. Clinton
clintondarleneM@uams.edu
PGY-1 Positions: 4
Required Research Year? No
Electives? No
http://www.uams.edu/ortho

California

Loma Linda University Program
Program Director: Montri D. Wongworawat, MD
Loma Linda University Medical Center
11406 Loma Linda Drive, Suite 218
Loma Linda, CA 92354
Tel: (909) 558-6444, ext. 62705
Residency Coordinator: Lora L. Benzatyan
lbenzatyan@llu.edu
PGY-1 Positions: 4
Required Research Year? No
Electives? No
http://www.lomalindaorthoresidency.org

Los Angeles County-Harbor-UCLA Medical Center Program
Program Director: Louis M. Kwong, MD
Los Angeles County-Harbor-UCLA Medical Center
1000 W Carson Street, Box 422
Torrance, CA 90509
Tel: (310) 222-2718
Residency Coordinator: Maria Garibay
magaribay@ladhs.org
PGY-1 Positions: 4
Required Research Year? No
Electives? No
http://www.harbor-ucla-ortho.org

Naval Medical Center (San Diego) Program
Program Director: Michael A. Thompson
Naval Medical Center
34800 Bob Wilson Drive, Suite 112
San Diego, CA 92134-5000
Tel: (619) 744-5332
Residency Coordinator: Lyn A. Martin
Ethyln.Martin@med.navy.mil
PGY-1 Positions: 5
Required Research Year? No
Electives? No
Note: Must be a member of the armed forces to participate in this program.
http://www.nmcsd.med.navy.mil

Saint Mary's Hospital and Medical Center Program
Program Director: William A. McGann, MD
Saint Mary's Medical Center
450 Stanyan Street
Orthopaedic Education Offices
San Francisco, CA 94117
Tel: (415) 750-5782
Residency Coordinator: Monica H. Bastidas
Monica.Bastidas@chw.edu
PGY-1 Positions: 3
Required Research Year? No
Electives? No
http://www.sforp.org

Stanford University Program
Program Director: James Gamble, MD
Stanford University Medical Center
Department of Orthopaedic Surgery
300 Pasteur Drive, Room R144
Stanford, CA 94305-5341
Tel: (650) 725-5903
Residency Coordinator: Karen Denny
kdenny@stanford.edu
PGY-1 Positions: 4
Note: An additional position is available at the PGY-2 level, and this resident will spend an additional year at the university hospital for a total of 5 years following internship.

Required Research Year? No
Electives? No
http://med.stanford.edu/shc/ortho

UCLA Medical Center Program
Program Director: James V. Luck Jr, MD
UCLA School of Medicine
10833 LeConte Ave, Room 72-225 CHS
Los Angeles, CA 90095-6902
Tel: (310) 825-6557
Residency Coordinator: Kathy Oka
koka@mednet.ucla.edu
PGY-1 Positions: 6
Required Research Year? No
Electives? No
http://ortho.ucla.edu

*University of California (Davis) Health
System Program*
Program Director: Rolando F. Roberto,
MD
University of California (Davis) Medical
Center
Department of Orthopaedic Surgery
4860 Y Street, Suite 3800
Sacramento, CA 95817
Tel: (916) 734-2807
Residency Coordinator: Loretta Adams
Loretta.adams@ucdmc.edu
PGY-1 Positions: 4
Required Research Year? No
Electives? Yes
http://www.ucdmc.ucdavis.edu/
orthopaedics

University of California (Irvine) Program
Program Director: Nitin N. Bhatia, MD
University of California Irvine Medical
Center
101 City Drive South
Departmentt of Orthopaedic Surgery
Pavillion III, 2nd Floor, Suite 81
Orange, CA 92868
Tel: (714) 456-5547
Residency Coordinator: Maria Guerrero
mlampino@uci.edu
PGY-1 Positions: 4
Required Research Year? No
Electives? Yes
http://www.orthopaedicsurgery.uci.edu

*University of California (San Diego)
Program*
Program Director: Alexandra K.
Schwartz, MD
UCSD Medical Center
350 Dickson Street, Mail Code 8894
San Diego, CA 92103-8894
Tel: (619) 543-7247
Residency Coordinator: Susan Driscoll
skdriscoll@ucsd.edu
PGY-1 Positions: 4
Required Research Year? Yes
Electives? Yes
http://www.ortho.ucsd.edu

*University of California (San Francisco)
Program*
Program Director: Thomas P. Vail, MD
UCSF Medical Center
Department of Orthopaedic Surgery
500 Parnassus Avenue, MU320W
San Francisco, CA 94143-0728
Tel: (415) 476-6043
Residency Coordinator: Delphean Quan
quand@orthosurg.ucsf.edu
PGY-1 Positions: 6
Required Research Year? No
Note: Applicants can apply for a 6-year
research track.
Electives? Yes
http://www.orthosurg.ucsf.edu

*University of Southern California/
LAC+USC Medical Center Program*
Program Director: David B.
Thorndarson, MD
University of Southern California School
of Medicine
2025 Zonal Avenue, GNH 3900
Los Angeles, CA 90033
Tel: (323) 226-7210
Residency Coordinator: Ruth Gomez
orthopod@usc.edu
PGY-1 Positions: 10
Required Research Year? No
Electives? Yes
http://www.usc.edu/medicine/
orthopaedic_surgery

Colorado

University of Colorado Denver Program
Program Director: Steven J. Morgan,
  MD
University of Colorado Health Sciences
  Center
12631 E. 17th Avenue
PO Box 6511, Mail Stop B-202
Denver, CO 80045
Tel: (303) 724-2961
Residency Coordinator: Mary M.
  Sampson
Mary.sampson@uchsc.edu
PGY-1 Positions: 4
Required Research Year? No
Electives? No
http://www.uchsc.edu/ortho

Connecticut

University of Connecticut Program
Program Director: Bruce D. Browner,
  MD
University of Connecticut Health Center
MARB 4th Floor
263 Farmington Avenue
Farmington, CT 06034
Tel: (860) 679-6640
Residency Coordinator: Virginia Cooper
Gcooper@nso.uchc.edu
PGY-1 Positions: 4
Required Research Year? No
Electives? No
http://www.uchc.edu

Yale–New Haven Medical Center Program
Program Director: Peter Jokl, MD
Yale-New Haven Hospital
PO Box 208071
New Haven, CT 06520
Tel: (203) 785-6907
Residency Coordinator: Katherine
  Umlauf
Kathryn.umlauf@yale.edu
PGY-1 Positions: 5
Required Research Year? No
Electives? No
http://medicine.yale.edu/ortho

District of Columbia

George Washington University Program
Program Director: Robert J. Neviaser,
  MD
George Washington University
2150 Pennsylvania Avenue NW, Room
  7-416
Washington, DC 20037
Tel: (202) 741-3311
Residency Coordinator: Ann Bond
abond@mfa.gwu.edu
PGY-1 Positions: 4
Required Research Year? No
Electives? No
http://www.gwumc.edu/edu/ortho

Georgetown University Program
Program Director: Sam W. Wiesel, MD
Georgetown University Hospital
Office of Education
Department of Orthopaedic Surgery
3800 Reservoir Road NW, G-PHC
Washington, DC 20007
Tel: (202) 444-7371
Residency Coordinator: Tori Leidel
vel1@gunet.georgetown.edu
PGY-1 Positions: 4
Required Research Year? No
Electives? No
http://www.georgetownuniversityhos-
  pital.org

Howard University Program
Program Director: Terry L. Thompson,
  MD
Howard University Hospital
Division of Orthopaedic Surgery
2041 Georgia Avenue NW
Washington, DC 20060
Tel: (202) 865-1656
Residency Coordinator: Sharon Britt
sdbritt@howard.edu
PGY-1 Positions: 4
Required Research Year? No
Electives? No
http://www.huhealthcare.com/gme/pro-
  grams.html

Florida

Jackson Memorial Hospital/Jackson Health System Program
Program Director: Frank J. Eismont, MD
Jackson Memorial Hospital
Rehabilitation Center, 3rd Floor, Room 303
1611 NW 12th Avenue
Miami, FL 33136
Tel: (305) 585-1315
Residency Coordinator: Carmen J. Fuente
cfuente@med.miami.edu
PGY-1 Positions: 7
Required Research Year? No
Electives? No
http://www.jhsmiami.org

Orlando Health Program
Program Director: Thomas A. Csencsitz, MD
Orlando Regional Medical Center
Medical Education—Orthopedics
22 West Underwood, 4th Floor
Orlando, FL 32806
Tel: (321) 841-1745
Residency Coordinator: Julie Brown
Julie.Brown@orhs.org
PGY-1 Positions: 4
Required Research Year? No
Electives? No
http://www.orlandohealth.com

University of Florida College of Medicine Jacksonville Program
Program Director: John S. Kirkpatrick, MD
University of Florida College of Medicine/Jacksonville
655 West 8th Street, ACC 2nd Floor, Box C126
Jacksonville, FL 32209
Tel: (904) 244-7757
Residency Coordinator: Patricia Edwards
Patricia.edwards@jax.ufl.edu
PGY-1 Positions: 4
Required Research Year? No
Electives? No
http://www.hscj.ufl.edu

University of Florida Program
Program Director: Mark Scarborough, MD
Department of Orthopaedics & Rehabilitation
PO Box 112727
Gainesville, FL 32611
Tel: (352) 273-7365
Residency Coordinator: Kendra Gallaugher
gallaks@ortho.ufl.edu
PGY-1 Positions: 4
Required Research Year? No
Electives? No
http://www.ortho.ufl.edu

University of South Florida Program
Program Director: G. Douglas Letson, MD
University of South Florida
Department of Orthopaedics
13220 USF Laurel Drive
MDF 5th Floor, MDC 106
Tampa, FL 33612
Tel: (813) 396-9639
Residency Coordinator: Ann Joyce
ajoyce@health.usf.edu
PGY-1 Positions: 4
Required Research Year? No
Electives: No
http://health.usf.edu/nocms/medicine/orthopaedic

Georgia

Atlanta Medical Center Program
Program Director: Steven M. Kane, MD
Atlanta Medical Center
303 Parkway Drive NE
PO Box 423
Atlanta, GA 30312
Tel: (404) 265-1579
Residency Coordinator: Marianna Watson
Marianna.Watson@tenethealth.com
PGY-1 Positions: 3
Required Research Year? No
Electives? No
http://www.atlantamedcenter.com

Dwight David Eisenhower Army Medical Center Program
Program Director: Russell A. Davidson, MD
Dwight David Eisenhower Army Medical Center
Orthopaedic Surgery Service
Fort Gordon, GA 30905
Tel: (706) 787-1859
Residency Coordinator: Jan Buff
Janie.buff@amedd.army.mil
PGY-1 Positions: 2
Required Research Year? No
Electives? No
Note: Must be enrolled in the armed forces to apply.
http://www.amedd.army.mil

Emory University Program
Program Director: Sherman V. Oskouei, MD
Emory University School of Medicine
Department of Orthopaedic Surgery
Residency Coordinator's Office, 315 ESOM Building
49 Jesse Hill Jr. Drive SE
Atlanta, GA 30303
Tel: (404) 778-1567
Residency Coordinator: Katherine Strozier
kstrozi@emory.edu
PGY-1 Positions: 5
Required Research Year? No
Electives? Yes
http://www.orthopaedics.emory.edu

Medical College of Georgia Program
Program Director: S. Marcus Fulcher, MD
Medical College of Georgia
Department of Orthopaedic Surgery
1120 15th Street
Augusta, GA 30912
Tel: (706) 721-1633
Residency Coordinator: Dorothy Harmon
dharmon@mcg.edu
PGY-1 Positions: 3
Required Research Year? No
Electives? No
http://www.mcg.edu

Hawaii

Tripler Army Medical Center Program
Program Director: Joseph R. Orchowski, MD
Tripler Army Medical Center
1 Jarrett White Road
Tripler AMC, HI 96859
Tel: (808) 433-3557
Residency Coordinator: Sherry Pico
Sherry.pico@us.army.mil
PGY-1 Positions: 3
Required Research Year? No
Electives? No
Note: Must be enrolled in the armed forces to apply.
http://www.tamc.amedd.army.mil

University of Hawaii Program
Program Director: Robert E. Atkinson, MD
University of Hawaii
John A. Burns School of Medicine
651 Ilalo Street
Honolulu, HI 96813
Tel: (808) 586-8234
Residency Coordinator: Gary Belcher
gbelcher@hawaii.edu
PGY-1 Positions: 2
Required Research Year? No
Electives? No
http://www.hawaiiresidency.org/orthopaedics/index.html

Illinois

Loyola University Program
Program Director: William J. Hopkins, MD
Loyola University Medical Center
2160 S. First Avenue
Maguire Building 105, Room 1700
Maywood, IL 60153
Tel: (708) 216-6906
Residency Coordinator: Rina Goslawski
cgoslawski@lumc.edu
PGY-1 Positions: 5
Required Research Year? No
Electives? No
http://www.stritch.luc.edu/depts/ortho/index.htm

McGaw Medical Center of Northwestern University Program
Program Director: Michael F. Schafer, MD
Northwestern University Feinberg School of Medicine
676 North Street Clair, Suite 1350
Chicago, IL 60611
Tel: (312) 926-4485
Residency Coordinator: Joan C. Broholm
j-broholm@northwestern.edu
PGY-1 Positions: 9
Required Research Year? No
Electives? No
http://www.orthopaedics.northwestern.edu

Rush University Medical Center Program
Program Director: Walter W. Virkus, MD
Rush University Medical Center
1653 West Congress Parkway, Room 1471 Jelke
Chicago, IL 60612
Tel: (312) 942-5850
Residency Coordinator: Beverly J. Kendall-Morgan
Beverly_Kendall-Morgan@rush.edu
PGY-1 Positions: 5
Required Research Year? No
Electives? No
http://www.rush.edu/gme

Southern Illinois University Program
Program Director: Keith R. Gabriel, MD
Southern Illinois School of Medicine
Division of Orthopaedics
PO Box 19679
Springfield, IL 62794-9679
Tel: (217) 545-6155
Residency Coordinator: Anita Weinhoeft
Aweinhoeft@siumed.edu
PGY-1 Positions: 3
Required Research Year? No
Electives? No
http://www.siumed.edu/surgery/orthopaedics

University of Chicago Program
Program Director: Brian C. Toolan, MD
University of Chicago Medical Center
5841 South Maryland Avenue, MC 3079
Chicago, IL 60637
Tel: (773) 834-2858
Residency Coordinator: Janet Stirn
jstirn@surgery.bsd.uchicago.edu
PGY-1 Positions: 4
Required Research Year? No
Electives? No
http://surgery.uchicago.edu/specialties/orthopaedic

University of Illinois College of Medicine at Chicago Program
Program Director: Alfonso Mejia, MD
University of Illinois Hospital
835 S Wolcott Avenue, Room E-270, M/C 844
Chicago, IL 60612
Tel: (312) 996-9858
Residency Coordinator: Theresa Mora
Tmora@uic.edu
PGY-1 Positions: 7
Required Research Year? No
Electives? No
http://chicago.medicine.uic.edu/departments___programs/departments/ortho

Indiana

Indiana University School of Medicine Program
Program Director: Randall T. Loder, MD
Indiana University Medical Center
541 Clinical Drive, Room 600
Indianapolis, IN 46202
Tel: (317) 274-3291
Residency Coordinator: Donna Roberts
Danders@iupui.edu
PGY-1 Positions: 5
Required Research Year? No
Electives? No
http://www.orthopaedics.iu.edu

Iowa

University of Iowa Hospitals and Clinics Program
Program Director: J. Lawrence Marsh, MD
University of Iowa Hospitals and Clinics
Orthopaedic Surgery
200 Hawkins Drive
Iowa City, IA 52242
Tel: (319) 356-2595
Residency Coordinator: Jeanette Marsh
Jeanette-marsh@uiowa.edu
PGY-1 Positions: 6
Required Research Year? No
Electives? No
http://www.uihealthcare.com/depts/
    med/orthopaedicsurgery/index.html

Kansas

University of Kansas School of Medicine Program
Program Director: Kimberly J. Templeton
University of Kansas Medical Center
Mail Stop 3017
3901Rainbow Boulevard
Kansas City, KS 66160
Tel: (913) 588-7590
Residency Coordinator: Janice Brunks
Jbrunks@kumc.edu
PGY-1 Positions: 4
Required Research Year? No
Electives? No
http://www2.kumc.edu/ortho

University of Kansas (Wichita) Program
Program Director: David McQueen, MD
University of Kansas School of Medicine Wichita
Orthopaedic Residency Program
929 North Street Francis, Room 4076
Wichita, KS 67214
Tel: (316) 268-5988
Residency Coordinator: Juanita E. Ridgeway
Jridgewa@kumc.edu
PGY-1 Positions: 4
Required Research Year? No
Electives? Yes
http://wichita.kumc.edu/ortho

Kentucky

University of Kentucky Medical Center Program
Program Director: William O. Shaffer, MD
Kentucky Clinic
740 S Limestone, K401
Lexington, KY 40536
Tel: (859) 218-3044
Residency Coordinator: Pauline Mills
Pmills@pop.uky.edu
PGY-1 Positions: 4
Required Research Year? No
Electives? No
http://www.mc.uky.edu/orthopaedics

University of Louisville Program
Program Director: Craig S. Roberts, MD
University of Louisville
Department of Orthopaedic Surgery
210 E Gray Street, Suite 1003
Louisville, KY 40202
Tel: (502) 852-6902
Residency Coordinator: Cheri Bingham
Cmbing02@gwise.louisville.edu
PGY-1 Positions: 4
Required Research Year? No
Electives? No
http://louisville.edu/medschool/
    orthopaedics

Louisiana

Louisiana State University Program
Program Director: Peter C. Krause, MD
Louisiana State University Health Sciences Center
Department of Orthopaedic Surgery
2025 Gravier Street, Room 330, Corridor J
New Orleans, LA 70112
Tel: (504) 568-4680
Residency Coordinator: Linda Flot
lflot@lsuhsc.edu
PGY-1 Positions: 4
Required Research Year? No
Electives? No
http://www.lsuhsc.edu

Louisiana State University (Shreveport) Program
Program Director: Margaret L. Olmedo, MD
Louisiana State University Health Sciences Center
1501 Kings Highway
PO Box 33932
Shreveport, LA 71130
Tel: (318) 675-4313
Residency Coordinator: Sylvia Carter
Scarte1@lsuhsc.edu
PGY-1 Positions: 3
Required Research Year? No
Electives? No
http://www.lsuhscshreveport.edu

Ochsner Clinic Foundation Program
Program Director: Mark S. Meyer, MD
Ochsner Clinic Foundation
1516 Jefferson Highway, 5th Floor, AT
New Orleans, LA 70121
Tel: (504) 842-5932
Residency Coordinator: Seimone Gilbert
segilbert@ochsner.org
PGY-1 Positions: 2
Required Research Year? No
Electives? No
http://www.ochsner.org

Tulane University Program
Program Director: John A. Davis Jr, MD
Tulane University Health Sciences Center
1430 Tulane Avenue, SL 32
New Orleans, LA 70112
Tel: (504) 988-5192
Residency Coordinator: Linda Miller
Limiller@tulane.edu
PGY-1 Positions: 2
Required Research Year? No
Electives? No
http://www.tulaneorthopaedics.com

Maryland

Johns Hopkins University Program
Program Director: Dawn LaPorte, MD
Johns Hopkins Orthopaedic Surgery
601 N Caroline Street, Suite 5223
Baltimore, MD 21287
Tel: (410) 955-8344
Residency Coordinator: Vicky Norton
Vnorton1@jhmi.edu
PGY-1 Positions: 5
Required Research Year? No
Electives? No
http://www.hopkinsortho.org

National Capital Consortium Program
Program Director: Patricia L. McKay, MD
National Naval Medical Center
Orthopaedic Surgery Service
8901 Wisconsin Avenue
Bethesda, MD 20889
Tel: (310) 319-4196
Residency Coordinator: Alice Anderson
Alice.anderson@med.navy.mil
PGY-1 Positions: 6
Required Research Year? Yes
Electives? No
http://www.bethesda.med.navy.mil

Union Memorial Hospital Program
Program Director: Leslie S. Matthews, MD
Union Memorial Hospital
201 East University Parkway
Baltimore, MD 21218
Tel: (410) 554-2857
Residency Coordinator: Kathy Lind
kathy.lind@medstar.net
PGY-1 Positions: 2
Required Research Year? No
Electives? No
http://www.unionmemorial.org

University of Maryland Program
Program Director: Robert S. Sterling, MD
University of Maryland School of Medicine
22 South Greene Street, Suite S11B
Baltimore, MD 21201
Tel: (410) 328-8915
Residency Coordinator: Nanette Catterton
ncatterton@umoa.umm.edu
PGY-1 Positions: 5
Required Research Year? No
Electives? No
http://www.umm.edu/orthopaedic

Massachusetts

Boston University Medical Center
Program
Program Director: Paul Tornetta, MD
Boston University Medical Center
850 Harrison Avenue, Dowling 2 North
Boston, MA 02118
Tel: (617) 638-8934
Residency Coordinator: Lynnette St.
Louis
Lynnette.stlouis@bmc.org
PGY-1 Positions: 5
Required Research Year? No
Electives? No
http://www.bumc.bu.edu/orthopaedics

*Massachusetts General Hospital/Brigham
and Women's Hospital/Harvard
Medical School Program*
Program Director: Dempsey Springfield,
MD
Massachusetts General Hospital
55 Fruit Street, WHT 535
Boston, MA 02114
Tel: (617) 726-2942
Residency Coordinator: Diane Sheehan
dsheehan@partners.org
PGY-1 Positions: 12
Required Research? No
Electives? No
http://www.hms.harvard.edu/ortho

Tufts Medical Center Program
Program Director: Charles Cassidy, MD
Tuft Medical Center
Department of Orthopedics, Box 306
800 Washington Street
Boston, MA 02111
Tel: (617) 636-5172
Residency Coordinator: Jane B. Dolph
Jdolph@tuftsmedicalcenter.org
PGY-1 Positions: 4
Required Research Year? No
Electives? No
http://www.tuftsmedicalcenter.org

University of Massachusetts Program
Program Director: Thomas F. Breen, MD
University of Massachusetts Medical
School
55 Lake Avenue North

Worcester, MA 01655
Tel: (508) 856-4262
Residency Coordinator: Michelle Auger
Michelle.auger@umassmed.edu
PGY-1 Positions: 4
Required Research Year? No
Electives? No
http://www.umassmed.edu/orthopedics

Michigan

Detroit Medical Center Program
Program Director: Ralph B. Baiser, MD,
JD
Sinai-Grace Hospital
Department of Orthopaedic Surgery
6071 West Outer Drive
Detroit, MI 48235
Tel: (313) 966-4750
Residency Coordinator: Kristen Stanley
kcooper@dmc.org
PGY-1 Positions: 4
Required Research? No
Electives? No
http://www.dmc.org/gme

*Grand Rapids Medical Education and
Research Center/Michigan State
University Program*
Program Director: David Rispler, MD
Grand Rapids Medical Education and
Research Center/Michigan State
University
Orthopaedic Residency Program
300 Lafayette, SE #3400
Grand Rapids, MI 49503
Tel: (616) 685-6615
tutschc@trinity-health.org
PGY-1 Positions: 5
Required Research Year? No
Electives? Yes
http://www.grmerc.net/ortho

Henry Ford Hospital Program
Program Director: Theodore W. Parsons
III, MD
Henry Ford Hospital
2799 West Grand Boulevard
Detroit, MI 48202
Tel: (313) 916-7520
Residency Coordinator: Kathleen Derrig
kderrig1@hfhs.org

PGY-1 Positions: 6
Required Research Year? No
Electives? No
http://www.henryford.com

*Kalamazoo Center for Medical Studies/
Michigan State University Program*
Program Director: Dale E. Rowe, MD
Kalamazoo Center for Medical Studies
Michigan State University
1000 Oakland Drive
Kalamazoo, MI 49008
Tel: (269) 337-6554
Residency Coordinator: Jennifer Austad
austad@kcms.msu.edu
PGY-1 Positions: 3
Required Research Year? No
Electives? Yes
http://www.kcms.msu.edu/orthopaedic-
surgery

McLaren Regional Medical Center Program
Program Director: Norman E. Walter,
MD
McLaren Regional Medical Center
Attn: Orthopedic Education Office
401 South Ballenger Highway
Flint, MI 48532
Tel: (810) 342-2111
Residency Coordinator: Rita Kotzian
ritak@mclaren.org
PGY-1 Positions: 2
Required Research Year? No
Electives? No
http://www.mclaren.org

University of Michigan Program
Program Director: Paul Dougherty, MD
University of Michigan Health System
1500 E Medical Center Drive, 2912D
    Taubman Center
Ann Arbor, MI 48109
Tel: (734) 232-6343
Residency Coordinator: Kelly Fearer
kfearer@med.umich.edu
PGY-1 Positions: 6
Required Research Year? No
Electives? No
http://www.med.umich.edu/ortho/edu/
res.htm

William Beaumont Hospital Program
Program Director: Harry N. Herkowitz,
MD
William Beaumont Hospital
3535 Thirteen Mile Road, Suite 744
Detroit, MI 48073
Tel: (248) 551-3140
Residency Coordinator: Lisa Thompson
Lthompson@beaumonthospitals.com
PGY-1 Positions: 5
Required Research Year? No
Electives? No
https://www.beaumonthospitals.com/
gme

Minnesota

*College of Medicine, Mayo Clinic
(Rochester) Program*
Program Director: Arlen D. Hanssen,
MD
Mayo School of Graduate Medical
Education
200 First Street SW
Rochester, MN 55905
Tel: (507) 284-3316
Residency Coordinator: Natalie Price
Price.Natalie@mayo.edu
PGY-1 Positions: 12
Required Research Year? No
Electives? No
http://www.mayo.edu/msgme

University of Minnesota Program
Program Director: Ann Van Heest, MD
University of Minnesota
Department of Orthopaedic Surgery
2450 Riverside Avenue S, R200
Minneapolis, MN 55454
Tel: (612) 273-8043
Residency Coordinator: Betsy
    Wehrwein
Wehrw005@umn.edu
PGY-1 Positions: 8
Required Research Year? No
Electives? No
http://www.ortho.umn.edu

Mississippi

University of Mississippi Medical Center Program
Program Director: Robert A. McGuire, MD
University of Mississippi Medical Center
2500 North State Street
Jackson, MS 39216
Tel: (601) 984-5153
Residency Coordinator: Susan Alexander
Salexander@orthopedics.umsmed.edu
PGY-1 Positions: 4
Required Research Year? No
Electives? Yes
http://orthopedics.umc.edu

Missouri

Saint Louis University School of Medicine Program
Program Director: Berton R. Moed, MD
Saint Louis University School of Medicine
Department of Orthopedic Surgery
3635 Vista Avenue at Grand Boulevard
St. Louis, MO 63110
Tel: (314) 577-8850
Residency Coordinator: Janel Britton
brittonj@slu.edu
PGY-1 Positions: 4
Required Research Year? Yes
Electives? No
http://orthopedics.slu.edu

University of Missouri at Kansas City Program
Program Director: James J. Hamilton, MD
University of Missouri-Kansas City
Department of Orthopaedic Surgery
2301 Holmes Street
Kansas City, MO 64108
Tel: (816) 556-3561
Residency Coordinator: Carolyn Holtman
Carolyn.holtman@tmcmed.org
PGY-1 Positions: 4
Required Research Year? No
Electives? No
http://www.med.umkc.edu/education

University of Missouri–Columbia Program
Program Director: Barry J. Gainor, MD
University of Missouri Columbia School of Medicine
One Hospital Drive, MC 213
Columbia, MO 65212
Tel: (573) 882-5731
Residency Coordinator: Sherri Boland
bolands@health.missouri.edu
PGY-1 Positions: 5
Required Research Year? No
Electives? No
http://som.missouri.edu/ortho

Washington University/B–JH/SLCH Consortium Program
Program Director: Rick W. Wright, MD
Barnes-Jewish Hospital
Orthopedic Surgery, Campus Box 8233
660 South Euclid Avenue
St. Louis, MO 63110
Tel: (314) 747-2835
Residency Coordinator: Michelle Tuetken
tuetkenm@wudosis.wustl.edu
PGY-1 Positions: 6
Required Research Year? No
Electives? No
http://www.ortho.wustl.edu

Nebraska

University of Nebraska Medical Center College of Medicine/Creighton University Program
Program Director: Matthew A. Mormino, MD
University of Nebraska Medical Center
Department of Orthopaedic Surgery
981080 Nebraska Medical Center
Omaha, NE 68198
Tel: (402) 559-2258
Residency Coordinator: Gerianne Miller
gmiller@unmc.edu
PGY-1 Position: 4
Required Research Year? No
Electives? No
http://www.unmcphysicians.com/ttg-ortho/new

New Hampshire

Dartmouth-Hitchcock Medical Center Program
Program Director: Charles F. Carr, MD
Dartmouth-Hitchcock Medical Center
One Medical Center Drive
Lebanon, NH 03756
Tel: (603) 653-6014
Residency Coordinator: Megan Linn
Megan.c.linn@hitchcock.org
PGY-1 Positions: 4
Required Research Year? No
Electives? No
http://www.dhmc.org/ortho

New Jersey

Monmouth Medical Center Program
Program Director: Steve J. Paragioudakis, MD
Monmouth Medical Center
300 Second Avenue
Long Branch, NJ 07740
Tel: (732) 923-6784
Residency Coordinator: Christine Steinberger
csteinberger@sbhcs.com
PGY-1 Positions: 2
Required Research Year? No
Electives? No
http://www.saintbarnabas.com/education

Seton Hall University School of Health and Medical Sciences Program
Program Director: Vincent K. McInerney, MD
Seton Hall University School of Graduate Medical Education
St Joseph's Regional Medical Center
703 Main Street
Paterson, NJ 07503
Tel: (973) 754-2926
Residency Coordinator: Catherine Riva
rivac@sjhmc.org
PGY-1 Positions: 3
Required Research Year? No
Electives? No
http://www.shu.edu/academics/grad-meded/orthopedic-surgery-residency/index.cfm

UMDNJ-New Jersey Medical School Program
Program Director: Joseph Benevenia, MD
UMDNJ-New Jersey Medical School
90 Bergen Street, Suite 7300
Newark, NJ 07101
Tel: (973) 972-3860
Residency Coordinator: Marie Birthwright
birthwma@umdnj.edu
PGY-1 Positions: 6
Required Research Year? No
Electives? No
http://njms.umdnj.edu/departments/orthopaedics/residency/index.cfm

UMDNJ-Robert Wood Johnson Medical School Program
Program Director: Charles J. Gatt, MD
UMDNJ-Robert Wood Johnson Medical School
51 French Street
PO Box 19
New Brunswick, NJ 08903
Tel: (732) 235-7869
Residency Coordinator: Eleanor Kehoe
kehoeem@umdnj.edu
PGY-1 Positions: 4
Required Research Year? No
Electives? No
http://rwjms2.umdnj.edu/orthoweb

New Mexico

University of New Mexico Program
Program Director: Robert Quinn, MD
Department of Orthopaedics & Rehabilitation
MSC10 5600
1 University of New Mexico
Albuquerque, NM 87131
Tel: (505) 272-6472
Residency Coordinator: Joni Roberts
jroberts@salud.unm.edu
PGY-1 Positions: 5
Required Research Year? No
Electives? No
http://hsc.unm.edu/som/ortho/index.shtml

New York

Albany Medical Center Program
Program Director: Richard L. Uhl, MD
Department of Orthopaedic Surgery
  Academic Office
1367 Washington Avenue, Suite 202
Albany, NY 12206
Tel: (518) 453-3079
Residency Coordinator: Kathy Pangburn
pangbuk@mail.amc.edu
PGY-1 Positions: 4
Required Research Year? No
Electives? No
http://www.amc.edu

Albert Einstein College of Medicine Program
Program Director: I. Martin Levy, MD
Montefiore Medical Center
1695 Eastchester Road, 2nd Floor
Bronx, NY 10461
Tel: (718) 405-8332
Residency Coordinator: Donna Chinea
dchinea@montefiore.org
PGY-1 Positions: 6
Required Research Year? No
Electives? No
http://www.einsteinortho.com

Hospital for Special Surgery/Cornell
  Medical Center Program
Program Director: Mathias P. Bostrom,
  MD
Hospital for Special Surgery
535 E 70th Street
New York, NY 10021
Tel: (212) 606-1466
Residency Coordinator: Pamela Sanchez
academictraining@hss.edu
PGY-1 Positions: 8
Required Research Year? No
Electives? No
http://www.hss.edu

Kingsbrook Jewish Medical Center Program
Program Director: Eli Bryk, MD
Kingsbrook Jewish Medical Center
585 Schenectady Avenue
Brooklyn, NY 11203-1891
Tel: (718) 604-5483
Residency Coordinator: Marlene Jackson
mjackson@kingsbrook.org
PGY-1 Positions: 1
Required Research Year? No
Electives? No
Note: Position only available to those
  applicants who have or will be finish-
  ing a preliminary general surgery year.
http://www.kingsbrook.org

Lenox Hill Hospital Program
Program Director: Elliot Hershman, MD
Lenox Hill Hospital
130 E 77th Street, 11th Floor
New York, NY 10075
Tel: (212) 434-2710
Residency Coordinator: Patricia
  Kennemur
pkennemur@lenoxhill.net
PGY-1 Positions: 2
Required Research Year? No
Electives? No
http://www.lenoxhillhospital.org

Maimonides Medical Center Program
Program Director: Jack Choueka, MD
Maimonides Medical Center
4802 Tenth Avenue
Brooklyn, NY 11219
Tel: (718) 283-8805
Residency Coordinator: Joanne Rotunno
jrotunno@maimonidesmed.org
PGY-1 Positions: 2
Required Research Year? Yes; 1 of 2
  residents enter a year of research after
  their PGY-2 year
Electives? No
http://www.maimonidesmed.org

Mount Sinai School of Medicine Program
Program Director: Bradford O. Parsons,
  MD
Mount Sinai Medical Center
One Gustave L Levy Place, Box 1188
New York, NY 10029
Tel: (212) 241-1621
Residency Coordinator: Amanda Mercado
amanda.mercado@mountsinai.org
PGY-1 Positions: 3
Required Research Year? No
Electives? No
http://www.mssm.edu/orthopaedics

New York Medical College at Westchester
Medical Center Program
Program Director: David E. Asprinio,
MD
New York Medical College at
Westchester Medical Center
95 Grasslands Road, Macy Pavilion
Room 008
Valhalla, NY 10595
Tel: (914) 493-8473
Residency Coordinator: Jean Aubel
aubelj@wcmc.com
PGY-1 Positions: 3
Required Research Year? No
Electives? No
http://www.nymc.edu

New York Medical College (Manhattan)
Program
Program Director: John R. Denton, MD
St. Vincent's Hospital Manhattan
170 West 12th Street, Spellman 7
New York, NY 10011
Tel: (212) 604-2502
Residency Coordinator: Barbara Piacente
bpiacente@svcmcny.org
PGY-1 Positions: 3
Required Research Year? No
Electives? No
http://www.svmortho.org

New York Presbyterian Hospital (Columbia
Campus) Program
Program Director: William N. Levine,
MD
Columbia University College of
Physicians & Surgeons
Department of Orthopedic Surgery
622 West 168th Street, Room PH11
New York, NY 10032
Tel: (212) 305-5974
Residency Coordinator: Ann Bravo-
Garcia
ab1308@columbia.edu
PGY-1 Positions: 6
Required Research Year? No
Electives? No
http://ps.cpmc.columbia.edu/electives/
Ortho1.html

New York University School of Medicine/
Hospital for Joint Diseases Program
Program Director: Kenneth A. Egol, MD
NYU-Hospital for Joint Diseases
301 East 17th Street, Room 1402
New York, NY 10003
Tel: (212) 598-6509
Residency Coordinator: Randie Godette
randie.godette@nyumc.org
PGY-1 Positions: 12
Required Research Year? Yes; 2 of 12
residents enter the lab after PGY-2
year.
Electives? No
http://www.med.nyu.edu/orthosurgery/
education/residency

NSLIJHS-Albert Einstein College of
Medicine at Long Island Jewish
Medical Center Program
Program Director: Nicholas A.
Sgaglione, MD
Long Island Jewish Medical Center
270-05 76th Avenue
New Hyde Park, NY 11040
Tel: (718) 470-7901
Residency Coordinator: Janice Vetrano
jvetrano@lij.edu
PGY-1 Positions: 3
Required Research Year? No
Electives? No
http://www.northshorelij.com

St. Luke's-Roosevelt Hospital Center
Program
Program Director: George L. Unis, MD
St. Luke's-Roosevelt Hospital Center
1111 Amsterdam Avenue, Clark 7, Room
5-703
New York, NY 10025
Tel: (212) 523-2650
Residency Coordinator: Christella Watts
cwatts@chpnet.org
PGY-1 Positions: 3
Required Research Year? No
Electives? No
http://www.wehealny.org

SUNY at Stony Brook Program
Program Director: James Penna, MD
Stony Brook University Hospital
Department of Orthopaedics
HSC T-18, Room 089
Stony Brook, NY 11794-8181
Tel: (631) 444-1487
Residency Coordinator: Gayle Siegel
gayle.siegel@sunysb.edu
PGY-1 Positions: 5
Required Research Year? No
Electives? No
http://www.stonybrookmedicalcenter.
   org/healthsciences

SUNY Health Science Center at Brooklyn
   Program
Program Director: William P. Urban Jr,
   MD
SUNY Health Science Center at
   Brooklyn
450 Clarkson Avenue, Box 30
Brooklyn, NY 11203
Tel: (718) 270-8995
Residency Coordinator: James Darrow
james.darrow@downstate.edu
PGY-1 Positions: 6
Required Research Year? No
Electives? No
http://www.downstate.edu

SUNY Upstate Medical University
   Program
Program Director: Stephen Albanese,
   MD
SUNY Health Science Center-Syracuse
Department of Orthopedic Surgery
750 East Adams Street
Syracuse, NY 13210
Tel: (315) 464-5226
Residency Coordinator: Julie Bordeau
bordeauj@upstate.edu
PGY-1 Positions: 4
Required Research Year? No
Electives? No
http://www.upstate.edu/ortho

University at Buffalo Program
Program Director: Lawrence B. Bone,
   MD
Erie County Medical Center

Department of Orthopaedic Surgery
462 Grider Street
Buffalo, NY 14215
Tel: (716) 898-5053
Residency Coordinator: Tammy Smith
tsmith4@buffalo.edu
PGY-1 Positions: 4
Required Research Year? No
Electives? No
http://wings.buffalo.edu/smbs/GME

University of Rochester Program
Program Director: C. McCollister Evarts,
   MD
University of Rochester Medical Center
601 Elmwood Avenue, Box 665
Rochester, NY 14642
Tel: (585)275-5168
Residency Coordinator: Karen Balta
Karen_balta@urmc.rochester.edu
PGY-1 Positions: 6
Required Research Year? No
Electives? No
http://www.urmc.rochester.edu/ortho

North Carolina

Carolinas Medical Center Program
Program Director: Steven L. Frick, MD
Carolinas HealthCare System
1616 Scott Avenue
PO Box 32861
Charlotte, NC 28203
Tel: (704) 355-3184
Residency Coordinator: Sherry Weeks
sherill.weeks@carolinashealthcare.org
PGY-1 Positions: 3
Required Research Year? No
Electives? No
http://www.carolinashealthcare.org

Duke University Program
Program Director: William T. Hardaker,
   MD
Duke University Medical Center
Division of Orthopaedic Surgery, Box
   3956
Durham, NC 27710
Tel: (919) 684-3170
Residency Coordinator: Wendy
   Thompson

wendy.thompson@duke.edu
PGY-1 Positions: 8
Required Research Year? No
Electives? No
http://orthoresidency.surgery.duke.edu

*University of North Carolina Hospitals
Program*
Program Director: Edmund R. Campion,
MD
University of North Carolina School of
Medicine
3144 Bioinformatics, CB 7055
Chapel Hill, NC 27599
Tel: (919) 966-9071
Residency Coordinator: Karen Gilliam
karen_gilliam@med.unc.edu
PGY-1 Positions: 5
Required Research Year? No
Electives? No
http://www.med.unc.edu/ortho

*Wake Forest University School of Medicine
Program*
Program Director: Ethan R. Wiesler,
MD
Wake Forest University School of
Medicine
Department of Orthopaedic Surgery
Medical Center Blvd, Box 1070
Winston-Salem, NC 27157
Tel: (336) 716-3946
Residency Coordinator: Kathleen
Hermance
hermance@wfubmc.edu
PGY-1 Positions: 4
Required Research Year? No
Electives? No
http://www.wfubmc.edu/ortho

Ohio

*Akron General Medical Center/
NEOUCOM Program*
Program Director: Mark C. Leeson, MD
Akron General Medical Center
400 Wabash Avenue, 224/430
Akron, OH 44307
Tel: (330) 344-6055
Residency Coordinator: Kathy Walsh
kwalsh@agmc.org

PGY-1 Positions: 3
Required Research Year? No
Electives? Yes
http://www.akrongeneral.org

Cleveland Clinic Foundation Program
Program Director: Thomas E. Kuivila,
MD
Cleveland Clinic Foundation
Department of Orthopaedic Surgery
9500 Euclid Avenue, A41
Cleveland, OH 44195
Tel: (216) 445-7570
Residency Coordinator: Christine
Orlinski
orlinsc@ccf.org
PGY-1 Positions: 6
Required Research Year? No
Electives? Yes
http://my.clevelandclinic.org

Mount Carmel Program
Program Director: Richard A.
Fankhauser, MD
Mount Carmel Health System
793 West State Street
Columbus, OH 43222
Tel: (614) 234-5354
Residency Coordinator: Lori Cropper
lcropper@mchs.org
PGY-1 Positions: 2
Required Research Year? No
Electives? Yes
http://www.mountcarmelhealth.com

Ohio State University Hospital Program
Program Director: Laura Phieffer, MD
Ohio State University Hospital
Department of Orthopaedics
N1050 Doan Hall
410 West 10th Avenue
Columbus, OH 43210
Tel: (614) 293-6194
Residency Coordinator: Julia Panzo
Panzo.6@osu.edu
PGY-1 Positions: 6
Required Research Year? No
Electives? No
http://www.ortho.ohio-state.edu

Summa Health System/NEOUCOM Program
Program Director: Jeffrey T. Junko, MD
Summa Health System
444 North Main Street
Akron, OH 44309-2090
Tel: (330) 379-5681
Residency Coordinator: Penny LaBate
labatep@summa-health.org
PGY-1 Positions: 3
Required Research Year? No
Electives? Yes
http://meded.summahealth.org

University Hospital/University of Cincinnati College of Medicine Program
Program Director: Keith Kenter, MD
University of Cincinnati Medical Center
231 Albert Sabin Way
PO Box 670212
Cincinnati, OH 45267
Tel: (513) 558-4592
Residency Coordinator: Kim Weingartner
weingaka@ucmail.uc.edu
PGY-1 Positions: 5
Required Research Year? No
Electives? No
http://www.med.uc.edu/ortho

University Hospitals Case Medical Center Program
Program Director: Randall E. Marcus, MD
University Hospitals of Cleveland–Case Medical Center
11100 Euclid Ave
Cleveland, OH 44106
Tel: (216) 844-3233
Residency Coordinator: Ellen Greenberger
egreenberger@msn.com
PGY-1 Positions: 6
Required Research Year? No
Electives? No
http://www.uhhospitals.org

University of Toledo Program
Program Director: Nabil A. Ebraheim, MD
University of Toledo-Health Science Campus

3065 Arlington Avenue
Suite, 2435
Toledo, OH 43614
Tel: (419) 383-6236
Residency Coordinator: Danielle Peace
danielle.peace@utoledo.edu
PGY-1 Positions: 4
Required Research Year? No
Electives? Yes
http://www.utoledo.edu/hscerror.html

Wright State University Program
Program Director: Richard T. Laughlin, MD
Wright State University Boonshoft SOM
30 E Apple Street, Suite 2200
Dayton, OH 45409
Tel: (937) 208-2127
Residency Coordinator: Peggy Baldwin
pkbaldwin@mvh.org
PGY-1 Positions: 4
Required Research Year? No
Electives? Yes
http://www.med.wright.edu/ortho/res

Oklahoma

University of Oklahoma Health Sciences Center Program
Program Director: Charles B. Pasque, MD
University of Oklahoma Health Sciences Center
PO Box 26901, Suite WP-1380
Oklahoma City, OK 73126
Tel: (405) 271-5964
Residency Coordinator: Janet Moore
Janet-moore@ouhsc.edu
PGY-1 Positions: 5
Required Research Year? No
Electives? No
http://www.oumedicine.com/academic-template_landing.cfm?id=2954

Oregon

Oregon Health & Science University Program
Program Director: Robert A. Hart, MD
Oregon Health & Science University
Mail Code Ortho – OP-31
3181 SW Sam Jackson Park Road

Portland, OR 97239
Tel: (503) 494-5842
Residency Coordinator: Pamela
  Feidelson
PGY-1 Positions: 2
Note: An additional position is offered
  outside of NRMP match.
Required Research Year? No
Electives? No
http://www.ohsu.edu

Pennsylvania

*Albert Einstein Healthcare Network
  Program*
Program Director: Eric A. Williams, MD
Albert Einstein Medical Center
5501 Old York Road, WCB4
Philadelphia, PA 19141
Tel: (215) 456-6051
Residency Coordinator: Stella Pietrzak
pietrzas@einstein.edu
PGY-1 Positions: 3; 2 of the 3 are avail-
  able through the NRMP match, 1 is
  offered outside of the match.
Required Research Year? No
Electives? No
http://www.einstein.edu

Allegheny General Hospital Program
Program Director: Mark E. Baratz, MD
Allegheny General Hospital
1307 Federal Street
Pittsburgh, PA 15212
Tel: (412) 359-6501
Residency Coordinator: Patricia Olzak
polzak@wpahs.org
PGY-1 Positions: 3
Required Research Year? No
Electives? No
http://www.wpahs.org

*Drexel University College of Medicine/
  Hahnemann University Hospital
  Program*
Program Director: Stephen J. Bosacco,
  MD
Drexel University College of Medicine
245 N 15th Street, Mail Stop 420
Philadelphia, PA 19102

Tel: (215) 762-8168
Residency Coordinator: Sandra Erby
serby@drexelmed.edu
PGY-1 Positions: 4
Required Research Year? No
Electives? No
http://www.drexelmed.edu

Geisinger Health System Program
Program Director: Gerald Cush, MD
Geisinger Medical Center
Department of Orthopaedic Surgery
100 N Academy Avenue
Danville, PA 17822
Tel: (570) 271-5555, ext 54033
Residency Coordinator: Jessica Temple
orthores@geisinger.edu
PGY-1 Positions: 2
Required Research Year? No
Electives? Yes
http://www.geisinger.edu

Hamot Medical Center Program
Program Director: John D. Lubahn, MD
Hamot Medical Center
201 State Street
Erie, PA 16550
Tel: (814) 877-6257
Residency Coordinator: Patricia J. Rogers
pat.rogers@hamot.org
PGY-1 Positions: 3
Required Research Year? No
Electives? No
http://www.hamot.org

*Penn State University/Milton S. Hershey
  Medical Center Program*
Program Director: Paul J. Juliano, MD
Milton S. Hershey Medical Center
Penn State Orthopedics, MC H089
30 Hope Drive, Building A, EC089
Hershey, PA 17033
Tel: (717) 531-4833
Residency Coordinator: Janice Woodley
jwoodley@hmc.psu.edu
PGY-1 Positions: 5
Required Research Year? No
Electives? No
http://www.pennstatehershey.org/web/
  orth

St. Luke's Hospital Program
Program Director: William G. DeLong Jr., MD
St. Luke's Hospital
801 Ostrum Street
Bethlehem, PA 18015
Tel: (610) 954-2369
Residency Coordinator: Erin McCartney
mccarte@slhn.org
PGY-1 Positions: 2
Required Research Year? No
Electives? No
http://www.mystlukesonline.org

Temple University Hospital Program
Program Director: Joseph J. Thoder, MD
Temple University Hospital
Broad & Ontario Streets
3401 N Broad Street
Philadelphia, PA 19140
Tel: (215) 707-8331
Residency Coordinator: Marianne Kilbride
marianne.killbride@tuhs.temple.edu
PGY-1 Positions: 4
Required Research Year? No
Electives? No
http://www.temple.edu/medicine

Thomas Jefferson University Program
Program Director: James J. Purtill, MD
Jefferson Medical College
1015 Walnut Street
Room 801, Curtis Building
Philadelphia, PA 19107
Tel: (215) 955-1500
Residency Coordinator: Susan Randolph
susan.randolph@jefferson.edu
PGY-1 Positions: 6
Required Research Year? No
Electives? No
http://www.tjuhortho.org

University of Pennsylvania Program
Program Director: Richard D. Lackman, MD
Hospital of University of Pennsylvania
3400 Spruce Street
2 Silverstein
Philadelphia, PA 19104
Tel: (215) 349-8731

Residency Coordinator: Barbara Weinraub
barbara.weinraub@uphs.upenn.edu
PGY-1 Positions: 8
Required Research Year? No
Electives? No
http://www.uphs.upenn.edu/ortho

University of Pittsburgh Medical Center Medical Education Program
Program Director: Vincent F. Deeney, MD
University of Pittsburgh School of Medicine
3471 Fifth Avenue, Suite 1000
Pittsburgh, PA 15213
Tel: (412) 605-3262
Residency Coordinator: Roberta Moenich
moenichrj@upmc.edu
PGY-1 Positions: 8
Required Research Year? No
Electives? No
http://www.orthonet.pitt.edu

Puerto Rico

University of Puerto Rico Program
Program Director: Manuel Garcia-Ariz, MD
University of Puerto Rico Medical Sciences Campus
Department of Orthopedic Surgery
PO Box 365067
San Juan, PR 00936-5067
Tel: (787) 764-5095
Residency Coordinator: Nestor Ramos-Alconini, MD
clrivera@rcm.upr.edu
PGY-1 Positions: 4
Required Research Year? No
Electives? No
http://www.md.rcm.upr.edu/orthopedics

Rhode Island

Brown University Program
Program Director: Christopher DiGiovanni, MD
Rhode Island Hospital
593 Eddy Street
Coop 1st Floor
Providence, RI 02903

Tel: (401) 444-4030
Residency Coordinator: Suzanne
Swanson
sswanson@lifespan.org
PGY-1 Positions: 6
Required Research Year? Yes
Electives? No
http://biomed.brown.edu/orthopaedics

South Carolina

*Greenville Hospital System/University
of South Carolina School of Medicine
Program*
Program Director: Kyle J. Jeray, MD
Greenville Hospital System
Department of Orthopaedic Surgery
701 Grove Road, 2nd Floor Support
Tower
Greenville, SC 29605
Tel: (864) 455-7878
Residency Coordinator: M. Fran Nelson
fnelson@.ghs.org
PGY-1 Positions: 4
Required Research Year? No
Electives? Yes
http://www.ghs.org

*Medical University of South Carolina
Program*
Program Director: John A. Glasser, MD
Medical University of South Carolina
96 Jonathan Lucas Street, CSB 708
PO Box 250622
Charleston, SC 29425
Tel: (843) 792-0245
Residency Coordinator: Cassandra
Tucker
tucker@musc.edu
PGY-1 Positions: 3
Required Research Year? No
Electives? No
http://gme.musc.edu

*Palmetto Health/University of South
Carolina School of Medicine Program*
Program Director: David E. Koon, MD
Palmetto Health Richland
2 Medical Park, Suite 404
Columbia, SC 29203
Tel: (803) 434-6879

Residency Coordinator: Michele Wehunt
michelle.wehunt@uscmed.sc.edu
PGY-1 Positions: 2
Required Research Year? No
Electives? No
http://residency.palmettohealth.org

Tennessee

*University of Tennessee College of Medicine
at Chattanooga Program*
Program Director: William M. Tew, MD
University of Tennessee College of
Medicine
Department of Orthopaedic Surgery
975 E Third Street, Hospital Box 260
Chattanooga, TN 37403
Tel: (423) 778-9202
Residency Coordinator: Donna Gibson
donna.gibson@erlanger.org
PGY-1 Positions: 3
Required Research Year? No
Electives? No
http://www.utcomchatt.org

University of Tennessee Program
Program Director: David R. Richardson,
MD
Campbell Foundation-University of
Tennessee
1211 Union Avenue, Suite 510
Memphis, TN 38104
Tel: (901) 759-3275
Residency Coordinator: Susan Coffill
scoffill@utmem.edu
PGY-1 Positions: 8
Required Research Year? No
Electives? No
http://www.utmem.edu

Vanderbilt University Program
Program Director: Herbert S. Schwartz,
MD
Vanderbilt University Medical Center
MCE South Tower, Suite 4200
1215 21st Avenue South
Nashville, TN 37232-8774
Tel: (615) 936-0100
Residency Coordinator: Jennifer Pelfrey
jennifer.pelfrey@vanderbilt.edu
PGY-1 Positions: 5

Required Research Year? No
Electives? No
http://www.vanderbilthealth.com/
orthopaedics

Texas

Baylor College of Medicine Program
Program Director: John V. Marymont,
MD
Baylor College of Medicine
Department of Orthopedic Surgery
1709 Dryden Road, 12th Floor
Houston, TX 77030
Tel: (713) 986-7390
Residency Coordinator: Desi Griffin
design@bcm.edu
PGY-1 Positions: 5
Required Research Year? No
Electives? No
http://www.bcm.edu/gme

*John Peter Smith Hospital (Tarrant County
Hospital District) Program*
Program Director: Russell A. Wagner,
MD
John Peter Smith Hospital
1500 Main Street
Fort Worth, TX 76104
Tel: (817) 927-1370
Residency Coordinator: Mary Bryant
mbryant@jpshealthnetwork.org
PGY-1 Positions: 4
Required Research Year? No
Electives? No
http://www.jpshealthnetwork.org

*San Antonio Uniformed Services Health
Education Consortium (BAMC)
Program*
Program Director: Tad L. Gerlinger, MD
Brooke Army Medical Center
Orthopaedic Surgery Service
3851 Roger Brooke Drive
Fort Sam Houston, TX 78234
Tel: (210) 916-3410
Residency Coordinator: Juanita Rogers
Juanita.magettrogers@amedd.army.mil
PGY-1 Positions: 4
Required Research Year? No
Electives? No

Note: Must be in the armed forces to
apply or have been accepted for a
HPSP scholarship.
http://www.sammc.amedd.army.mil

*San Antonio Uniformed Services Health
Education Consortium (WHMC)
Program*
Program Director: Craig R. Ruder, MD
Wilford Hall Medical Center/SGOYV
2200 Bergquist Drive, Suite 1
Lackland AFB, TX 78236
Tel: (210) 292-5875
Residency Coordinator: Wanda Williams
wanda.williams@lackland.af.mil
PGY-1 Positions: 4
Required Research Year? No
Electives? No
Note: Must be in the armed forces/Air
Force to apply.
http://www.whmc.af.mil

*Texas A&M College of Medicine-Scott and
White Program*
Program Director: Mark D. Rahm, MD
Scott and White Memorial Hospital
2401 South 31st Street
Temple, TX 76508
Tel: (254) 724-5455
Residency Coordinator: Mary McKeown
mmckeown@swmail.sw.org
PGY-1 Positions: 4
Required Research Year? No
Electives? No
http://www.sw.org

Texas Tech University (Lubbock) Program
Program Director: George W. Brindley,
MD
Texas Tech University Health Sciences
Center
3601 4th Street Stop 9436
Lubbock, TX 79430
Tel: (806) 743-1704
Residency Coordinator: Christy Morrison
christy.morrison@ttuhsc.edu
PGY-1 Positions: 3
Required Research Year? No
Electives? No
http://www.ttuhsc.edu/som/ortho

University of Texas at Houston Program
Program Director: William C. McGarvey, MD
University of Texas Medical School at Houston
6431 Fannin, MSB 6.142
Houston , TX 77030-1501
Tel: (713) 500-7012
Residency Coordinator: Kristey Tedder
kristey.tedder@uth.tmc.edu
PGY-1 Positions: 3
Required Research Year? No
Electives? No
http://med.uth.tmc.edu

University of Texas Health Science Center at San Antonio Program
Program Director: Daniel W. Carlisle, MD
University of Texas Health Science Center
7703 Floyd Curl Drive
San Antonio, TX 78229
Tel: (210) 567-5139
Residency Coordinator: Theresa Hill
hillt@uthscsa.edu
PGY-1 Positions: 6
Required Research Year? No
Electives? No
http://www.uthscsa.edu/orthopaedics

University of Texas Southwestern Medical School Program
Program Director: Joseph Borrelli Jr., MD
University of Texas Southwestern Medical Center
5323 Harry Hines Boulevard
Dallas, TX 75390
Tel: (214) 645-3143
Residency Coordinator: Menyon Menefee
menyon.menefee@utsouthwestern.edu
PGY-1 Positions: 6
Required Research Year? No
Electives? No
http://www.utsouthwestern.edu

University of Texas Medical Branch Hospitals Program
Program Director: Kelly D. Carmichael, MD
University of Texas Medical Branch
301 University Boulevard
Galveston, TX 77555
Tel: (409) 747-5727
Residency Coordinator: Kathy Flesher
kflesher@utmb.edu
PGY-1 Positions: 5
Required Research Year? No
Electives? No
http://www.utmb.edu/ortho

William Beaumont Army Medical Center/Texas Tech University (El Paso) Program
Program Director: Philip J. Belmont Jr, MD
William Beaumont Army Medical Center
5005 North Piedras Street
El Paso, TX 79920-5001
Tel: (915) 569-2288
Residency Coordinator: Freda Fry
Freda.fry@amedd.army.mil
PGY-1 Positions: 4
Required Research Year? No
Electives? No
Note: Must be a member of the armed forces to participate in this program.
http://www.wbamc.amedd.army.mil

Utah

University of Utah Program
Program Director: Alan Stotts, MD
University of Utah Orthopedic Center
590 Wakara Way
Salt Lake City, UT 84108
Tel: (801) 587-5448
Residency Coordinator: Elise Collins
Elise.collins@hsc.utah.edu
PGY-1 Positions: 5
Required Research Year? No
Electives? No
http://www.med.utah.edu/orthopedics

Vermont

University of Vermont Program
Program Director: S. Elizabeth Ames, MD
University of Vermont College of Medicine
Department of Orthopaedics and Rehabilitation
440 Stafford Building
Burlington, VT 05405
Tel: (802) 656-2250
Residency Coordinator: Melissa Gara
melissa.kretmar@uvm.edu
PGY-1 Positions: 3
Required Research Year? No
Electives? No
http://www.med.uvm.edu/ortho

Virginia

Naval Medical Center (Portsmouth) Program
Program Director: Robert T. Ruland, MD
Naval Medical Center
620 John Paul Jones Circle
27 Effingham Street
Portsmouth, VA 23708
Tel: (757) 953-1814
Residency Coordinator: Kelley Jacobson
kelly.jacobson@med.navy.mil
PGY-1 Positions: 4
Required Research Year? No
Electives? No
Note: Must be a member of the armed forces to participate in this program.
http://www.med.navy.mil/SITES/NMCP/Pages/default.aspx

University of Virginia Program
Program Director: Bobby Chhabra, MD
University of Virginia Health System
PO Box 800159
Charlottesville, VA 22908
Tel: (434) 243-0265
Residency Coordinator: Mindy Franke
mcf3f@virginia.edu
PGY-1 Positions: 5
Required Research Year? No
Electives? No
http://www.healthsystem.virginia.edu

Virginia Commonwealth University Health System Program
Program Director: Wilhelm A. Zueler, MD
Medical College of Virginia
Department of Orthopaedic Surgery
1200 East Broad Street
PO Box 980153
Richmond, VA 23298
Tel: (804) 827-1204
Residency Coordinator: Amber Cox
orthoresprog@vcu.edu
PGY-1 Positions: 5
Required Research Year? No
Electives? No
http://www.vcu.edu/orthopaedics

Washington

Madigan Army Medical Center Program
Program Director: Edward D. Arrington, MD
Madigan Army Medical Center
Attn: MCHJ-SOP
Orthopedic Surgery Service
Tacoma, WA 98431
Tel: (253) 968-0167
Residency Coordinator: Jan Sanders
jan.sanders@us.army.mil
PGY-1 Positions: 3
Required Research Year? No
Electives? No
Note: Must be part of the armed forces to participate in this program.
http://www.mamc.amedd.army.mil

University of Washington Program
Program Director: Douglas P. Hanel, MD
University of Washington
Department of Orthopedics
Campus Box 354743
4245 Roosevelt Way NE, Suite E110
Seattle, WA 98105
Tel: (206) 598-9960
Residency Coordinator: Angela Weiss
amweiss@u.washington.edu
PGY-1 Positions: 8
Required Research Year? No
Electives? No
http://www.orthop.washington.edu

West Virginia

Marshall University School of Medicine Program
Program Director: Ali Oliashirazi, MD
Marshall University School of Medicine
1600 Medical Center Drive, Suite G-500
Huntington, WV 25701-3655
Tel: (304) 691-1149
Residency Coordinator: Deborah Adkins
muortho@marshall.edu
PGY-1 Positions: 3
Required Research Year? No
Electives? No
http://musom.marshall.edu

West Virginia University Program
Program Director: Sanford E. Emery, MD
West Virginia University
Department of Orthopaedics
PO Box 9196
Morgantown, WV 26506
Tel: (304) 293-1168
Residency Coordinator: Cindy Thompson
cthompson@hsc.wvu.edu
PGY-1 Positions: 3
Required Research Year? No
Electives? No
http://www.hsc.wvu.edu/som/ortho

Wisconsin

Medical College of Wisconsin Affiliated Hospitals Program
Program Director: Gregory J. Schmeling, MD
MCW Clinics @FMLH East
MCW Orthopaedics
9200 West Wisconsin Avenue
Milwaukee, WI 53226
Tel: (414) 257-7399
Residency Coordinator: Anne Kinowski
akinowski@mcw.edu
PGY-1 Positions: 5
Required Research Year? No
Electives? No
http://www.mcw.edu/ortho

University of Wisconsin Program
Program Director: Matthew W. Squire, MD
University of Wisconsin Hospital and Clinics
K/7 Clinical Science Center
600 Highland Avenue
Madison, WI 53792
Tel: (608) 263-0888
Residency Coordinator: Leigh Larson
larson@ortho.wisc.edu
PGY-1 Positions: 5
Required Research Year? No
Electives? No
http://www.orthorehab.wisc.edu

Sample Personal Statements

SAMPLE PERSONAL STATEMENT FOR AN ORTHOPEDIC RESIDENCY 1

I would like to pursue a residency in orthopedic surgery because it is a unique and gratifying specialty in which surgeons are able to cure many of the musculoskeletal conditions of their patients. I believe that my unconventional path from working in finance to pursuing a career in medicine as well as my experiences in orthopedic research make me a unique and well-qualified candidate.

I worked as a financial analyst on the corporate derivatives sales and trading desk at JP Morgan for 3 years prior to pursuing a career in medicine. As an analyst, I often worked together on a team with professionals from different departments within the investment bank to develop financial solutions for corporations. After being promoted to associate, I led client meetings, developed corporate relationships, and trained and mentored new analysts and interns to develop a strong team and individual work ethic. Teamwork is essential to accomplish the complex task of structuring and implementing derivative products to manage the financial risks of large multinational corporations. I have learned from my orthopedic rotations during medical school that both teamwork and leadership are essential to running a successful surgical service. As a resident, I will strive to apply and further develop these skills to ensure high-quality patient care.

In addition to becoming a productive member of my future residency program, I am also very interested in orthopedic research. I participated in the Bones Hospital Summer Fellowship during my first summer of medical school and worked with an orthopedic surgeon. I not only gained exposure to clinical orthopedics by shadowing him during office hours and assisting in operating room procedures, but I also performed biomechanical research. I evaluated the tensile strength of rotator cuff repair sutures on a sheep tendon model. My research was sponsored in part by a grant from the Chinese American Medical Society, and I presented my project at their Annual Scientific Meeting in the fall of 2005. This project gave me a glimpse of the exciting opportunities for investigation and advancement in the practice of orthopedics.

During that summer, I also began a clinical research study to examine the early complications of proximal humerus fractures treated with locked plates. I developed the research protocol and obtained IRB approval at several Bones Hospital-affiliated institutions. I have continued to work on this project during the past 2 years, gathering and analyzing physical exam and radiographic data. My research has been presented as a podium presentation at the American Academy of Orthopedic Surgeons Annual Meeting in February 2007, as a poster at the Orthopedic Trauma Association Annual Conference in October 2006, and a manuscript was recently submitted to the *Journal of Orthopedic Trauma*. This experience has been extremely rewarding and has shown me the exciting opportunities to contribute to the development of orthopedics through research as well as the satisfaction of being a clinician and treating patients.

I believe that my past experiences prior to and during medical school have taught me valuable lessons that can be applied to a career in orthopedic surgery. It is my hope to train at a residency program that will provide me with a comprehensive foundation of knowledge in all of the different areas of orthopedics as well as opportunities in research. My ultimate goal is to obtain the best training available so that I may become a skilled orthopedic surgeon and also contribute to further developments in the field through research.

Comments: The strong points of this statement are (1) it gives the reader an idea of the applicant's personality; (2) it emphasizes work/research experiences; (3) it explains why the applicant is interested in orthopedics; (4) it describes what the applicant wants to achieve during residency; and (5) it defines the applicant's long-term goals.

SAMPLE PERSONAL STATEMENT FOR AN ORTHOPEDIC RESIDENCY 2

I thoroughly enjoyed my third year of medical school—released into the hospital, able to help patients and work with the house staff. I found the hospital to be a communal environment with people working toward the collective goal of patient care. In that context, there were many fields that interested me, so it was not until the end of my surgical clerkship that I determined that orthopedics was my field of choice. Apart from the visceral thrill of the procedures and enjoyment of interacting with the orthopedic team, I am drawn to orthopedics for many reasons.

Orthopedics works to preserve patients' quality of life by restoring their physical functioning. One's identity is often influenced by his or her level of mobility and independence. Being fortunate enough to have all 4 surviving grandparents, I have seen how various orthopedic interventions have been able to keep them mobile and independent into, and through, their 80s. As the average life expectancy increases, the demand on orthopedics to aid in the maintenance of an independent, able-bodied population is increasing as well. This is a challenge the field seems prepared to face. Intimately connected with technology, the practice of orthopedics is constantly evolving. Innovations in techniques and materials both improve patient care as well as ensure a continually evolving and interesting practice throughout a long career.

I am also drawn to orthopedics for it utilizes both surgical and non-surgical treatment modalities, giving the physician a diverse range of treatment options. This enables the orthopedic physician to help patients with various degrees of disability and to work with them over a continued course of treatment. I look forward to these longitudinal patient relationships, for it is the patient that makes medicine interesting and rewarding. In my early career, I have experienced this first hand. During my medicine clerkship, I worked closely with a patient who suffered from CMV encephalitis. He had become demented and was subsequently restrained for weeks. As a result, some of the hospital staff had come to interact with this patient on a merely cursory level. I was bothered by the limited attention afforded to this patient. Optimistic his prognosis could improve with increased attention and effort, I spent additional time with this patient, taking the initiative to improve the situation. I challenged him to walk around the hospital and was the catalyst for multiple radiation therapy appointments. Our activity together both hastened his physical rehabilitation and demonstrated the extent of his cognitive improvements, prompting the caregiving team to engage the patient in a more comprehensive and compassionate manner, thereby promoting his recovery. This experience was a strong affirmation of my natural optimism and comfort with taking the initiative. It demonstrated the benefits of taking personal responsibility for patient care and working through the inertia that can result from difficult situations.

Patient care initially attracted me to the field of medicine, and through my clinical experience, I have learned specifically how I wish to practice. As a proactive and optimistic person, I am drawn to orthopedics for it offers an exciting combination of concrete problem solving, evolving technology, intense patient care, and professional camaraderie. I am inspired to work hard and with dedication—characteristics with which I am familiar. Diagnosed with dyslexia in elementary school, I went on to be a writing tutor for my peers in college. This is indicative of years of working longer and harder than my colleagues, initially to keep up and then to excel. From this experience and others, I have come to enjoy the challenges and the rewards of hard work. I look forward to an orthopedic residency as the next invigorating challenge.

Comments: Although this statement does not talk about work/research experience, it attracts the reader on a more personal level. The strong points of this statement are (1) it gives the reader an idea of the applicant's personality; (2) it describes the applicant's dedication and how it is relevant to orthopedics; (3) it describes personal experiences/struggles that may not have been conveyed elsewhere in the student's application; and (4) it explains why the applicant is interested in orthopedics.

SAMPLE PERSONAL STATEMENT FOR AN ORTHOPEDIC FELLOWSHIP 1

My interest in adult reconstructive surgery began during medical school and has increased through both clinical and research exposures during my residency training. I have found that the improvements in the quality of life offered by total joint arthroplasty are unparalleled, and the sense of satisfaction afforded by working with these patients is immense.

As part of a 1-year research fellowship during my residency, I became involved with projects utilizing molecular biology investigative techniques and also became intimately involved with clinical projects examining periprosthetic infection, thromboembolism, clinical outcomes of implants, and perioperative blood utilization. These endeavors have been among the most rewarding parts of my residency training. I have 3 main goals for a fellowship in adult reconstructive surgery. My first goal is to become proficient in complex primary and revision total hip and knee arthroplasty. As adult reconstructive surgery enters its fifth decade, and as total joint arthroplasty is increasingly performed in younger patients, the number of revision procedures performed is certain to increase in the future. As an adult reconstructive surgeon, I feel it is crucial to be able to tackle the most complex cases, and a fellowship will expose me to the advanced operative techniques necessary to treat this patient population.

The second goal of my fellowship is to improve my skills in the planning, performance, and synthesis of research to prepare me for a career in academic orthopedic surgery. The final goal of my fellowship is to improve my ability to be an orthopedic educator in the clinic, in the operating room, and in the research lab.

My future goals include a career in academic orthopedic surgery as a specialist in adult reconstruction. I am attracted to the challenges provided by working in a referral center where the most complex problems are managed. I feel that the training of future physicians and orthopedic surgeons is among the greatest challenges and rewarding endeavors that a person can undertake, and I look forward to becoming more involved in research, teaching, and participation in professional societies in the future.

Comments: While the fellowship applicant's personal statement naturally reflects a greater range of experience and training than the residents', the core emphases are essentially the same, including work/research experiences, why the applicant is interested in adult reconstructive surgery, what the applicant hopes to achieve during the fellowship, and the applicant's long-term goals.

SAMPLE PERSONAL STATEMENT FOR AN ORTHOPEDIC FELLOWSHIP 2

After a broad exposure to the field of orthopedics during my first few years of residency, I found my genuine interests gravitating toward disorders and treatment of the upper extremity. Specifically, reading about the shoulder was pleasurable and not the necessary chore I felt with some other subjects. In addition, we are in the midst of understanding the natural history of many shoulder diseases and how we can potentially improve their outcomes. Our surgical and non-surgical interventions are rapidly evolving; it seems with each new journal issue, there is yet another, potentially better way to treat particular pathology. Thus, this is an exciting time for shoulder surgery.

My interest in elbow surgery differs from that related to the shoulder. I find the elbow to be more complex and occasionally intimidating to many orthopedists. That challenge piqued my interest, and I want to serve as a resource for a community that may otherwise struggle with complex fractures, overuse injuries, or arthritis. Beyond my particular interest in the shoulder and elbow anatomically, my personality suits a specialty where I can treat a full spectrum of injury or pathology.

I am specifically pursuing the fellowship at Bones Hospital because I feel that it will best prepare me for a future career as a shoulder and elbow subspecialist. My ideal fellowship includes extensive exposure to arthroscopic and open approaches, fracture work, and reconstructive surgery of both the shoulder *and* the elbow. Your program clearly excels in meeting these requirements. Also of interest to me is the opportunity to utilize ultrasound as a diagnostic tool.

The literature produced from your institution clearly illustrates progressive thinking and an attempt to answer significant questions that are clinically relevant. I want to learn in that environment so that I may treat my future patients by the most appropriate means and so that I may answer such questions in the future.

Comments: This statement shows a different approach that can be used. It is intended to be more personalized to specific programs. The applicant states why he is interested in shoulder and elbow surgery; why he is interested in and a good candidate for a specific program, and what he hopes to achieve during the fellowship; and the applicant's long-term goals.

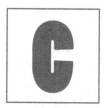

Sample Curriculum Vitae

Sample CV 1

Curriculum Vitae
Joseph Bones, BS

456 Main Street
Anytown, WI 53902
Home phone: (419) 555-1212
Work phone: (419) 555-2121

Date of Birth: 4/5/78
SSN: 777-45-1234
E-mail: drybones@hotmail.com

Education

Nuronz School of Medicine, Healthville, MN 74382
MD degree, expected 2010
United States Medical Licensing Examination Step I, 12/2001; Score: 250

Pacific State College
Daly City, CA 92345
BS, 2000, Major in Biochemistry

Work Experience

Manager: Dairy Queen, Anytown, WI
Summer 1996
Skills obtained included competency with the use of spreadsheets and electronic inventory systems

Publications

Domo M, Bones J. Hybrid total hip arthroplasty: a long-term follow-up study. *J Bone Joint Surg Am*. 1998;34:354-355.
Bones J. Why every residency program should want me. Scientific paper, presented at the American Academy of Orthopaedic Surgeons 1999 Annual Meeting, Anaheim, CA.

Research Experience

1. Honors Research: Histologic characterization of regenerate bone formed during distraction osteogenesis. December 1997–June 1999. Advisor: Orthopedic D. Chairman, MD

2. Bone Morphogenic Protein Project: Studying the effects of BMP injected intorat fractures. November 1997–April 1998. Advisor: Orthopedic D. Chairman, MD

Honors and Awards

Alpha Omega Alpha, elected September 1999
Raphe J. Zuzawa Award for Undergraduate Research, 1998

Extracurricular activities

Hiking, biking, golf

SAMPLE CV 2

John A. Bennett, BA

515 West Street
New York, NY 10016
(212) 222-3456, John.Bennett@gmail.com

Education

MD, Fracture School of Medicine, New York, NY
August 2003-May 2008

BS, Union College, Schenectady, NY
Major: Biology; September 1999-June 2003

Awards and Honors

Fracture School of Medicine

✓ 2006-2007	Research Scholar, National Institutes of Health Cloisters Research
	Scholars Program

Union College

✓ 2003	The Phi Beta Kappa Society
✓ 2003	Magna Cum Laude Graduate

Research Experience

7/2006-6/2007	Position: Research Scholar (National Institutes of Health
Topic:	Evaluation of the Potent Src Kinase Inhibitor AZD0530 in Metastatic Osteosarcoma Cell Lines and Animal Models)
Investigator:	Joe Wilson, DVM, PhD
	National Cancer Institute, National Institutes of Health

Related Experience

Summer 2004   Fracture University Department of Orthopedic Surgery
                       Summer
                       Externship Program

Extracurricular Activities

2004-2005   Co-President, Black and Latino Student Association
2004-2005   Co-Chapter President, Student National Medical Association

Publications

1. Bennett JA, Doe J. Case report: two step malignant transformation of a liposcleros-
    ing myxofibrous tumor of bone. *Clin Orthop Relat Res.* 2008;466:2873-2877.

2. Bennett JA. Analysis of the cross-sectional area of the adductor longus tendon:
    a descriptive anatomic study. *American Journal of Sports Medicine.* 2007;35:996-
    999.

Abstracts and Presentations

1. Bennett JA. Evaluation of the Potent Src Inhibitor AZD0530 in metastatic
    osteosarcoma cell lines. National Institutes of Health Cloisters Research Scholars
    Program Meeting, 2007 (Abstract).

2. Bennett JA. Inhibition of the metastatic potential of the osteosarcoma cell Lines by
    the Potent Src Inhibitor AZD0530. American Association for Cancer Research,
    2007 (Abstract).

Interests and Hobbies

Volunteering, mentoring children, playing basketball, weight lifting, music, reading,
    avid sports fan, socializing with family and friends.

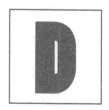

SAMPLE OPERATIVE REPORTS FOR COMMON ORTHOPEDIC PROCEDURES

The following operative reports are examples of write-ups for operative procedures of the sort that you can expect to perform during your residency.

SAMPLE OPERATIVE REPORT 1

PATIENT NAME:

MEDICAL RECORD NUMBER:

DATE OF PROCEDURE:

SURGEON:

FIRST ASSISTANT:

SERVICE: Orthopedic Surgery

ANESTHESIOLOGIST:

ANESTHESIA:

PREOPERATIVE DIAGNOSIS: Closed left tibia/fibula fracture with compartment syndrome.

POSTOPERATIVE DIAGNOSIS: Closed left segmental tibia and fibular fracture with 4-compartment syndrome, left leg.

PROCEDURE:
1. Four-compartment fasciotomies, left leg.
2. Open intramedullary fixation, left tibia fracture.

IMPLANTS USED: 10 x 380 tibial cannulated nail.

ESTIMATED BLOOD LOSS:

BLOOD REPLACED:

DRAINS:

SPECIMENS:

COMPLICATIONS:

INDICATION FOR SURGERY: The patient is a 27-year-old male involved in a pedestrian versus motor vehicle injury. He sustained a displaced closed left tibial shaft fracture. Shortly after admission, he developed paresthesias, compartments that were tense, as well as anterior blistering. He had pain with passive stretch of the toes. After the risk, benefits, and alternative of operative and non-operative treatment were discussed at length with the patient, he was brought to the operating room for 4-compartment fasciotomy and intramedullary fixation of the tibia.

PROCEDURE: After the induction of spinal anesthesia, the patient was given prophylactic intravenous antibiotics. After the patient's non-operative extremity was carefully positioned and secured to the operating room table, the left lower extremity was prepped and draped in the usual sterile fashion. Fasciotomy incisions were then carried out with the distal medial incision approximately 2 to 3 cm posterior to the posterior border of the tibia and the anterolateral incision proximally in the midline between the tibia and the fibula. The medial incision was carried out sharply. A branch of the saphenous vein was cauterized. Scissor dissection was used down to the fascia with visualization of the fascia over the soleus. This was divided longitudinally. There was moderate bulging noted; however, there was a significant amount of hematoma present underneath the fascia of the deep posterior compartment.

The fascia over the deep posterior compartment of the leg was then incised with removal of a large amount of hematoma. The neurovascular bundle was found to be intact. Laterally, the incision likewise was carried out, and the fascia was visualized. An H incision was made over the interval of the anterior and the lateral compartments with visualization of septum. Using scissors once again beneath the fascia, the lateral release was carried out first distally and then proximally followed by the anterior compartment release. There was found to be, again, moderate bulging of the muscle after the release with substantial muscular contusion noted. The superficial peroneal nerve was found to be intact in the lateral compartment.

With the completion of the fasciotomies, an incision was then made in the midline prepatellar area with a number 15 blade. Hemostasis was obtained with an electrocautery followed by blunt dissection of the subcutaneous tissues down to the ligamentum patella. A median parapatellar incision was carried out. The capsule was visualized. The retroligamentous fat pad was visualized and the proximal tibia palpated. Using a curved awl, a starting point was established, and appropriate alignment was confirmed on both AP and lateral plane using fluoroscopy. A ball-tipped guide wire was then inserted into the tibial shaft under image intensification. The fracture was then reduced, and while the reduction was held, the guide wire was advanced across the fracture site and distally to the physeal scar. With the guide wire seated, the length was then measured to 385 mm and a 380-mm nail was selected as the appropriate length. While the fracture reduction was maintained and with intermittent fluoroscopic control, the canal was then sequentially reamed in 0.5-mm increments from 8 mm to 11.5 mm, making the correct nail diameter to be 10 mm. The ball-tipped guide wire was then exchanged for a non–ball-tipped guide wire with an exchange tube, and appropriate placement was confirmed fluoroscopically. The nail was then gently inserted using a mallet, and appropriate reduction in AP and lateral planes was confirmed. The nail was then locked proximally with two bolts using the appropriate jig and distally with two bolts using a "perfect circle" technique. The wounds were irrigated at this point with sterile saline, and the locking screw sites were closed with staples. The median parapatellar incision was closed with 0, followed by inverted 2-0 sutures in the subcutaneous tissues and skin staples.

Wet-to-drys were applied to the fasciotomy sites. Final AP and lateral radiographs were obtained and confirmed acceptable fracture reduction and appropriate hardware placement. A long-leg splint was applied with the knee in extension. The patient was then returned to his bed and taken to the recovery room in stable condition.

POSTOP PLAN: The patient will be maintained on prophylactic intravenous antibiotics. His leg will be continually elevated, and he will return to the OR in 48 hours for repeat debridement of his fasciotomy sites followed by attempted delayed primary closure or split-thickness skin grafting.

Sample Operative Report 2

PATIENT NAME:

MEDICAL RECORD NUMBER:

DATE OF PROCEDURE:

SURGEON:

FIRST ASSISTANT:

SERVICE: Orthopedic Surgery

ANESTHESIOLOGIST:

ANESTHESIA:

PREOPERATIVE DIAGNOSES:
1. Right distal radius fracture.
2. Closed fracture of right third metacarpal.
3. Closed fracture of right fourth metacarpal.
4. Right carpal tunnel syndrome, acute.

POSTOPERATIVE DIAGNOSES:
1. Right distal radius fracture.
2. Closed fracture of right third metacarpal.
3. Closed fracture of right fourth metacarpal
4. Right carpal tunnel syndrome, acute.

OPERATION:
1. Open treatment, right third and fourth metacarpals with internal fixation.
2. Closed reduction, right distal radius.
3. Application of Uniplane external fixator, right wrist.
4. Open right carpal tunnel release.

ESTIMATED BLOOD LOSS:

BLOOD REPLACED:

DRAINS:

COMPLICATIONS:

FINDINGS:
1. Comminuted extra-articular right distal radius fracture.
2. Comminuted shaft fracture of the right third metacarpal.
3. Closed long spiral fracture of the right fourth metacarpal shaft.
4. Preoperative examination consistent with acute carpal tunnel syndrome.

SPECIMENS: None.

INDICATION FOR SURGERY: The patient is a 46-year-old male, manual laborer who fell approximately 30 feet off of a ladder. He was brought to Bones Hospital Trauma Center with the above-described injuries. In addition, he had a pneumothorax. He was cleared by the trauma team and subsequently brought to the operating room for fixation of his fractures. The risks and benefits of surgery were discussed with the patient before entering the operating room. All questions were answered.

PROCEDURE: After induction of axillary block anesthesia, the patient was placed supine on the operating room table. A tourniquet was placed proximally on the right upper extremity. The right upper extremity was prepped and draped in the usual sterile fashion. The arm was exsanguinated using an Esmarch bandage, and the tourniquet was inflated to 250 mmHg. A dorsal incision was made in the interspace between the third and fourth metacarpals on the dorsal aspect of the hand.

Dissection was carried down carefully through the subcutaneous tissue. The subcutaneous veins and sensory nerves were carefully protected. Incision was made in the fascia adjacent to the third metacarpal. The fracture was easily identified. Curets and freer elevator were used to clear soft tissue from the fracture lines. The fracture was held in reduction using reduction clamps. Two 1.5-mm lag screws were placed across the large butterfly fragment using standard lag screw technique. Excellent reduction was achieved. A 1.5-mm plate was cut to a 5-hole length and placed over the dorsal-radial aspect of the third metacarpal. Three screws were then placed proximally and three distally in the plate across both cortices of the metacarpal. Excellent purchase was achieved with all screws. Excellent reduction of the fracture was achieved. The fascia was then repaired over the metacarpal. Thorough irrigation was performed before closing this fascia.

Attention was then turned to the fourth metacarpal. An incision was made in the fascia overlying the fourth metacarpal. The periosteum was minimally elevated. This fracture configuration was a long spiral that extended two-thirds of the length of the metacarpal. The fracture ends were carefully cleared of all soft tissues. The fracture was held in reduction with two dental picks. A 1.5-mm lag screw was placed across these two fragments using standard lag screw technique. Excellent purchase was achieved with the screw, and excellent reduction of the fracture was achieved. Two additional lag screws were placed across the long spiral fragment. An attempt was made to place the lag screws in different planes to increase the mechanical strength of the construct. Intraoperative fluoroscopic imaging in two planes was performed to confirm excellent reduction of the fractures and good position of all implants. The wound was then thoroughly irrigated. The fascia overlying the fourth metacarpal was carefully repaired using interrupted 4-0 sutures.

The skin was closed using interrupted 4-0 nylon sutures. Because of the patient's preoperative carpal tunnel symptoms and the fact that he was having surgical intervention that would cause additional swelling, we proceeded with open carpal tunnel release. A 1.5-cm incision was made over the anterior aspect of the right hand at the base of the palm. Dissection was carried down carefully through the subcutaneous tissue. The palmar fascia was incised along the lines of the skin. The subcutaneous veins and sensory nerves were carefully protected. The transverse carpal ligament was identified. A small portion of the palmaris brevis was visualized and minimally disturbed. The transverse carpal ligament was incised under direct visualization.

The entire length of the transverse carpal ligament was incised. This was confirmed by visual inspection and gentle palpation with a Freer elevator. The median nerve was slightly compressed within the carpal tunnel, and there was immediate hyperemia after release of the transverse carpal ligament.

The wound was then thoroughly irrigated. The skin was closed using interrupted 4-0 nylon sutures.

Next, the external fixator was placed across the wrist. A dorsal-radial incision was made at the junction of the middle and distal thirds of the forearm. Dissection was carried down carefully through the subcutaneous tissue. The brachioradialis tendon was identified. The dorsal sensory branch of the radial nerve was identified emerging from underneath the brachioradialis. The ECRB and ECRL tendons were identified. The interval between the ECRL and ECRB tendons was identified. The periosteum over the radius was incised and elevated slightly to facilitate placement of the pins. Using the appropriate drill guides, three 3-mm pins were placed in the radius in the appropriate configuration. The wound was then thoroughly irrigated. The subcutaneous tissue was closed using 4-0 sutures. The skin was closed using a running 3-0 Prolene suture. Two small stab incisions were made over the dorsal-radial aspect of the right index metacarpal. A 3-mm pin was placed in the metacarpal through the stab wounds after cleaning soft tissue off of the bone. The tourniquet was released. Any bleeding vessels were cauterized using Bovie electrocautery. Fluoroscopic imaging in two planes was used to confirm excellent position of all pins. The pins in the radius were advanced slightly so that 1 to 2 threads protruded from the distal cortex. The position of the pins was determined to be in good position based on AP and lateral fluoroscopic images. The external fixator frame was assembled.

The fracture was reduced by closed means using longitudinal traction followed by slight palmar translation. The bolts were tightened on the external fixator. Fluoroscopic imaging was used to confirm excellent reduction of the extra-articular distal radius fracture with reconstitution of radial length, radial inclination, and restoration of palmar tilt to the distal radius on the lateral view to approximately neutral. The second bar of the external fixator frame was applied, and all bolts were tightened. Sterile dressings were applied. Intraoperative plain radiographs were taken to confirm excellent reduction of the fracture and position of all hardware. The patient was then brought to the recovery room in stable condition, having tolerated the procedure well.

SAMPLE OPERATIVE REPORT 3

PATIENT NAME:

MEDICAL RECORD NUMBER:

DATE OF PROCEDURE:

SURGEON:

FIRST ASSISTANT:

SERVICE: Orthopedic Surgery

ANESTHESIOLOGIST:

ANESTHESIA: General

PREOPERATIVE DIAGNOSIS: Closed left femur fracture.

POSTOPERATIVE DIAGNOSIS: Closed left femur fracture.

OPERATION: Intramedullary nail fixation of left femur fracture.

ESTIMATED BLOOD LOSS:

BLOOD REPLACED:

DRAINS:

COMPLICATIONS:

INDICATION FOR SURGERY: This 22-year-old female sustained a closed left femoral shaft fracture as a result of a motor vehicle crash last night. Surgery is indicated in order to restore length and alignment to the limb and to facilitate functional rehabilitation. We discussed the operative and non-operative treatment options as well as the relative risks and benefits of each with the patient. On our recommendation, she has agreed to proceed with surgical treatment. All questions were answered.

PROCEDURE: The patient was brought to the operating room and placed on the operating room table in the supine position where general anesthesia was induced and an oral endotracheal tube was passed. She was then turned to the right lateral decubitus position where bony prominences were well padded. The left lower extremity was then prepared and draped sterilely. We used fluoroscopy for assistance throughout the case. We passed a guide wire percutaneously through the skin proximally into the piriformis fossa. Position of the guide wire was then confirmed using biplanar fluoroscopy. An incision was made around the guide wire, and the soft tissues were spread. A 9-mm drill bit was then passed over the guide wire and used to enlarge the opening into the proximal femoral intramedullary canal. We passed the fracture reduction tool and a guide wire into the proximal femoral intramedullary canal and then, using biplanar fluoroscopy, reduced the fracture and passed the guide wire across the fracture site into the distal fragment. We prepared the femur for nailing by reaming. We started with a 9-mm endcutting reamer and progressed in 0.5-mm increments to 11.5 mm.

We measured the length of the femur using a guide wire and then selected a 40 cm x 10 mm diameter femoral nail. We loaded the nail onto the driving guide and then passed it over the guide wire, through the proximal fragment, across the fracture site, and into the distal fragment after the ball-tipped guide wire had been exchanged for a non–ball-tipped guide wire. We then removed the guide wire and proceeded with interlocking. We interlocked distally first. We used one distal interlocking screw. The more proximal of the two distal interlocking holes was chosen for fixation. The screw was placed using fluoroscopic assistance and a free-hand technique. No difficulty was encountered. We then attached the extraction device to the nail proximally and drove the nail retrograde approximately 2 to 3 mm to achieve compression across the fracture site.

We proceeded next with proximal interlocking. One proximal interlocking screw was placed from lateral to medial through a lateral stab incision. Fluoroscopic assistance and the proximal interlocking guide were used for assistance with placement of this screw. We next confirmed the position and alignment of the hardware and fracture fluoroscopically. All wounds were closed after copious irrigation using inverted 2-0 sutures in the subcutaneous tissues followed by skin staples. At this point, dry sterile dressings were applied to the wounds. The length and alignment of the leg were measured clinically and noted to be good. My plan for postoperative management is to allow weight-bearing as tolerated on the operated left lower extremity. The patient will receive 24 hours of postoperative prophylactic antibiotics.

Sample Operative Report 4

PATIENT NAME:

MEDICAL RECORD NUMBER:

DATE OF PROCEDURE:

SURGEON:

FIRST ASSISTANT:

SERVICE: Orthopedic Surgery

ANESTHESIOLOGIST:

ANESTHESIA: General

PREOPERATIVE DIAGNOSIS: Left tibial pilon fracture.

POSTOPERATIVE DIAGNOSIS: Left tibial pilon fracture.

OPERATION: Closed reduction with manipulation and multiplane external fixation of left pilon fracture.

ESTIMATED BLOOD LOSS:

BLOOD REPLACED:

DRAINS:

COMPLICATIONS:

INDICATION FOR SURGERY: The patient is a 41-year-old male status post severe injury to his left ankle. The patient was initially seen and noted to have a comminuted fracture of the distal tibia and associated fibula fracture (pilon fracture). The patient was seen in follow-up today in orthopedic clinic and noted to have severe soft tissue swelling fracture blisters and loss of reduction of his distal tibial fracture. Because of his poor reduction and status of his soft tissues, this patient was felt to be a candidate for external fixation to maintain length and gross alignment of his distal tibial fracture to allow his soft tissues to heal in preparation for open reduction, internal fixation. The risks versus benefits of the procedure were explained to the patient preoperatively. He stated he understood this and was in agreement with plans for treatment.

PROCEDURE: After induction of general endotracheal anesthesia, the left lower extremity was prepped and draped in sterile fashion. External fixation frame was constructed by placing three 5-mm half-pins in the midshaft of the tibia from anterior to medial direction. Two 4-mm transfixion pins were then placed in the calcaneus from a medial to lateral direction. Finally, two 4-mm half-pins were placed in the first metatarsal from a dorsal medial direction. A multiplane external fixation was then constructed maintaining the ankle in neutral dorsiflexion, maintaining the talus underneath the tibia and reasonable reduction of the distal tibia and fibular fractures.

Intraoperative fluoroscopy confirmed the reduction, and the frame was then tightened. The forefoot pins were then attached to the frame and used to maintain the forefoot in plantigrade nonsupinated position. Intraoperative x-rays revealed good position of the fracture and external fixator. Pin sites were then cleaned and dressed, and then Xeroform gauze was placed over the fracture blisters once they were debrided. The patient was then awakened and transferred to the recovery area in stable condition. Estimated blood loss was minimal. There were no drains and no complications.

The postoperative plan will be elevation, non–weight-bearing status, and delayed open reduction, internal fixation when the soft tissue status allows in 1 to 2 weeks.

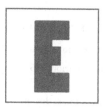

SAMPLE POSTOPERATIVE CHECKS FOR ORTHOPEDIC PATIENTS

The following postoperative order sets are designed to serve as a template for junior residents and medical students to aid them in writing their postop notes and ensure they do not miss anything vital in their assessment.

1. Postop check for right total knee replacement

S: Patient complains of mild right knee pain. Denies shortness of breath, chest pain, lightheadedness, or dizziness.

O: Tmax 100.3, Tcurrent 99.5, BP 130/75, HR 84, RR 18

RLE: Dressing: clean, dry, and intact

Motor: Dorsiflexors (Tibialis anterior) 5/5, Plantarflexors (Gastrocsoleus complex) 5/5
        Extensor Hallucis Longus (EHL) 5/5
        Sensation intact to light touch distally
        Vascular: DP pulse 2+, PT pulse 2+, cap refill <2 secs all toes
        Calves: soft, nontender bilaterally; foot pumps in place bilaterally
        Hemovac output: 100 cc/last 8 hours
        Postop H/H; 9.7/29.2

A/P: 74 y/o male S/P R TKR-stable postop.
        Check hemoglobin and hematocrit in am.
        Continuous passive motion (CPM) to right knee to begin in am.
        Monitor hemovac output. Continue intravenous antibiotics while hemovac in place.
        Aspirin and foot pumps for DVT prophylaxis.
        OOB in am with physical therapy.
        Encourage incentive spirometry.
        Continue intravenous PCA for pain relief.

2. Postop check for right total hip replacement

S: Patient c/o lightheadedness and dizziness. Denies chest pain or shortness of breath. Denies right hip pain.

0:	Tmax 100.7, Tcurrent 99.2, BP 100/60, HR 110, RR 16, 02 sat 97%
Right Hip:	Dressing: mild serosanguinous drainage noted
Motor:	Dorsiflexors (Tibialis Anterior) 5/5, Plantarflexors (Gastrocsoleus complex) 5/5, EHL 5/5
	Sensation intact to light touch distally
Vascular:	DP 2+, PT 2+, cap refill <2 secs
Calves:	Soft, nontender bilaterally.
	Abduction pillow in place.
	Foot pumps in place bilaterally.
Hemovac output:	120 cc/last 8 hours.
Postop H/H;	7.9/24.5
Postop EKG:	Sinus tachycardia at rate of 110, no ischemic changes.
A/P:	76 y/o male S/P R THR with postop anemia. Past medical history significant for hypertension. Preop H/H 9.9/32.5. Postop H/H 7.9/24.5. Patient c/o lightheadedness and dizziness. Denies shortness of breath or chest pain. Tachycardic to 110. BP 100/60. Two units autologous blood available.
Plan:	Will transfuse 1 unit autologous blood now. Will recheck H/H 1 hour after transfusion. Discussed transfusion with attending physician who agrees with current plan. Monitor vital signs.

Continue iron, folate, and colace. Also recheck CBC in am. Continue aspirin and foot pumps for DVT prophylaxis. Continue total hip precautions. Abduction pillow at all times. Monitor hemovac output. Will D/C hemovac when output <30 cc/8 hours. Continue IV antibiotics while hemovac in place. Continue morphine for pain relief. Physical and occupational therapy to start in am. Encourage incentive spirometry.

3. Postop check for open rotator cuff repair

S:	Patient without complaints. Denies numbness or tingling right upper extremity.
0:	Afebrile, vital signs stable (AF, VSS)
RUE:	Dressing: clean, dry, and intact
Motor:	Axillary (deltoid), Musculocutaneous (biceps), Radial (wrist extension) Ulnar (able to cross fingers), AIN (O-Kay sign), PIN (EPL), Median (thumb pinch) function intact 5/5.

Sensation intact to light touch axillary (deltoid patch on upper arm), musculocutaneous (lateral forearm), radial (dorsal web space between thumb and index finger), ulnar (distal ulnar aspect of little finger), median (distal radial aspect of index finger).

Vascular:	Radial pulse 2+, capillary refill <2 secs
A/P:	52 y/o M S/P open rotator cuff repair stable. Occupational therapy to start in am: PROM PFE 100, PER 30, IR to chest wall, no active ROM, Pendulum exercises.
	Prophylactic IV antibiotics x 24 hours.
	Likely discharge tomorrow after being seen by OT.

4. Postop check for anterior cervical discectomy and fusion (ACDF)

S: Patient without complaints. Denies difficulty breathing or shortness of breath.

0: Afebrile, BP 120/80, HR 82, RR 14

Neck: Philadelphia collar in place, primary dressing clean, dry, and intact

Motor: C5 (deltoid/biceps) 5/5, C6 (wrist extension) 5/5, C7 (wrist flexors, finger extension, triceps) 5/5, C8 (finger flexion, hand intrinsics) 5/5, TI (hand intrinsics) 5/5, L2 (iliopsoas) 5/5, L3 (quadriceps) 5/5, L4 (tibialis anterior) 5/5, L5 (extensor hallucis longus) 5/5, SI (gastrocsoleus complex) 5/5.

Sensation: C3 (upper anterior neck), C4 (lower anterior neck), C5 (lateral arm), C6 (lateral forearm), C7 (middle finger), C8 (medial forearm), TI (medial arm) intact to light touch LI (anterior superior iliac spine), L2 (anterior aspect of midthigh), L3 (anterior thigh above patella), L4 (m3edial leg and medial foot), L5 (lateral leg and dorsum of foot), SI (lateral foot) intact to light touch.

Vascular: Radial pulse 2+ bilaterally, dorsalis pedis 2+ bilaterally, posterior tibialis 2+ bilaterally. Capillary refill <1 second throughout.

Reflexes: Biceps (C5), Brachioradialis (C6), Triceps (C7) all present and symmetric. Patellar reflex (L4) and Achilles reflex (SI) present and symmetric. Negative Hoffman's bilaterally. Plantar response flexor bilaterally. No clonus.

Calves: Soft, nontender bilaterally. SCD boots in place bilaterally.

JP drain: 10 cc previous 8 hours. Postop Hg 11.0, Hct 35.9

A/P: 42 y/o male SIP anterior cervical discectomy and fusion C5-C6. Stable postop. Monitor neck for swelling. Continue SCD boots for DVT prophylaxis. Monitor JP output. Will likely D/C JP in am. Pain control. Encourage ambulation. PT/OT

5. Postop check for microlumbar discectomy

S: Patient complains of mild low back pain. Denies leg pain. Denies numbness or tingling. No other complaints.

0: Afebrile, VSS

Dsg: Clean, dry, and intact

Motor: L2 (iliopsoas) 5/5, L3 (quadriceps) 5/5, L4 (tibialis anterior) 5/5, L5 (extensor hallucis longus) 5/5, SI (gastrocsoleus complex) 5/5

Sensation: LI (ASIS), L2 (anterior aspect of midthigh), L3 (anterior thigh above patella), L4 (medial leg and medial foot), L5 (lateral leg and dorsum of foot), SI (lateral foot) sensation intact to light touch.

Vascular: DP 2+ bilaterally, PT 2+ bilaterally.

Reflexes: Patellar reflex (L4) present and symmetric. Achilles reflex (S1) present and symmetric.

Plantar response is flexor bilaterally. No clonus.

Calves: Soft, nontender bilaterally.
SCD boots in place bilaterally.
Postop Hg 10.9, Hct 34.0

A/P: 45 y/o F S/P microlumbar discectomy L5/S1 stable.
Will increase dose of subQ morphine for better pain control.
Monitor closely for respiratory depression.
Encourage OOB and incentive spirometer.
PT/OT for ambulation training in am.
SCD boots for DVT prophylaxis.
Continue current care.

6. Postop check for intramedullary nailing R closed tibia fracture

S: Patient without complaints.

0: AF, VSS

RLE: Dressing: clean, dry, intact. Splint in place.
DF 5/5, PF 5/5, EHL 5/5
Sensation intact to light touch L4-S I
DP 2+ , PT 2+ , capillary refill <2 secs throughout all toes
No pain on passive extension of toes

Calves: Soft, nontender bilaterally.

Postop Hg: 10.7, Hematocrit 34.0

A/P: 32 y/o M SIP intramedullary nailing R closed tibia fracture.
Stable postop.
Check CBC in am.
Lovenox for DVT prophylaxis.
PT/OT. WBAT.
Encourage OOB and ambulation.
Encourage incentive spirometry.

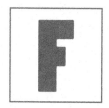

ONLINE EDUCATIONAL AIDS

American Academy of Orthopaedic Surgeons (AAOS)
www.aaos.org

American Orthopaedic Foot and Ankle Society (AOFAS)
www.aofas.org

American Orthopaedic Society of Sports Medicine (AOSSM)
www.sportsmed.org

American Shoulder and Elbow Surgeons (ASES)
www.ases-assn.org/web/index.html

American Society for Surgery of the Hand (ASSH)
www.assh.org

Arthroscopic Association of North America (AANA)
www.aana.org

North American Spine Society (NASS)
www.spine.org

OrthoGate
www.orthogate.org

Orthopaedic Trauma Association (OTA)
www.ota.org

Pediatric Orthopaedic Society of North America (POSNA)
www.posna.org

PubMed

www.ncbi.nlm.nih.gov/pubmed

VuMedi

www.vumedi.com

Wheeless's Textbook of Orthopaedics

www.wheelessonline.com

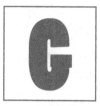

ACGME CORE COMPETENCIES

Residents will be regularly evaluated on the following 6 competencies, eventually achieving the expected level of a new practitioner. The pertinent information will be reviewed and compiled as part of the semi-annual review by the program director. Achievement of satisfactory performance levels for all 6 competencies will be necessary for successful completion of the program.

The residency program must require that its residents obtain competence in the 6 areas listed below to the level expected of a new practitioner. Programs must define the specific knowledge, skills, behaviors, and attitudes required and provide educational experiences as needed in order for their residents to demonstrate the following:

1. *Patient care* that is compassionate, appropriate, and effective for the treatment of health problems and the promotion of health. Residents are expected to:
   a. Communicate effectively and demonstrate caring and respectful behaviors when interacting with patients and their families
   b. Gather essential and accurate information about their patients
   c. Make informed decisions about diagnostic and therapeutic interventions based on patient information and preferences, up-to-date scientific evidence, and clinical judgment
   d. Develop and carry out patient management plans
   e. Counsel and educate patients and their families
   f. Demonstrate the ability to practice culturally competent medicine
   g. Use information technology to support patient care decisions and patient education
   h. Perform competently all medical and invasive procedures considered essential for the area of practice
   i. Provide health care services aimed at preventing health problems or maintaining health
   j. Work with health care professionals, including those from other disciplines, to provide patient-focused care

Information used with permission of the Accreditation Council for Graduate Medical Education © ACGME 2009

2. **Medical knowledge** about established and evolving biomedical, clinical, and cognate (eg, epidemiological and social-behavioral) sciences and the application of this knowledge to patient care. Residents are expected to:

   a. Demonstrate an investigatory and analytic thinking approach to clinical situations

   b. Know and apply the basic and clinically supportive sciences that are appropriate to their discipline

3. **Practice-based learning and improvement** that involves investigation and evaluation of their own patient care, appraisal and assimilation of scientific evidence, and improvements in patient care. Residents are expected to:

   a. Analyze practice experience and perform practice-based improvement activities using a systematic methodology

   b. Locate, appraise, and assimilate evidence from scientific studies related to their patients' health problems

   c. Obtain and use information about their own population of patients and the larger population from which their patients are drawn

   d. Apply knowledge of study designs and statistical methods to the appraisal of clinical studies and other information on diagnostic and therapeutic effectiveness

   e. Use information technology to manage information, access on-line medical information, and support their own education

   f. Facilitate the learning of students and other health care professionals

4. **Interpersonal and communication skills** that result in effective information exchange and collaboration with patients, their families, and other health professionals. Residents are expected to:

   a. Create and sustain a therapeutic and ethically sound relationship with patients

   b. Use effective listening skills and elicit and provide information using effective nonverbal, explanatory, questioning, and writing skills

   c. Work effectively with others as a member or leader of a health care team or other professional group

5. **Professionalism,** as manifested through a commitment to carrying out professional responsibilities, adherence to ethical principles, and sensitivity to a diverse patient population. Residents are expected to:

   a. Demonstrate respect, compassion, and integrity; a responsiveness to the needs of patients and society that supersedes self-interest; accountability to patients, society, and the profession; and a commitment to excellence and ongoing professional development

   b. Demonstrate a commitment to ethical principles pertaining to provision or withholding of clinical care, confidentiality of patient information, informed consent, and business practices

   c. Demonstrate sensitivity and responsiveness to patients' culture, age, gender, and disabilities

   d. Demonstrate sensitivity and responsiveness to fellow health care professionals' culture, age, gender, and disabilities

6. *Systems-based practice*, as manifested by actions that demonstrate an awareness of and responsiveness to the larger context and system of health care and the ability to effectively call on system resources to provide care that is of optimal value. Residents are expected to:

   a. Understand how their patient care and other professional practices affect other health care professionals, the health care organization, and the larger society and how these elements of the system affect their own practice

   b. Know how types of medical practice and delivery systems differ from one another, including methods of controlling health care costs and allocating resources

   c. Practice cost-effective health care and resources allocation that does not compromise quality of care

   d. Advocate for quality patient care and assist patients in dealing with system complexities

   e. Know how to partner with health care managers and health care procedures to assess, coordinate, and improve health care and know how these activities can affect system performance

**Please refer to http://www.acgme.org/acWebsite/RRC_260/SSVproject/SVR-Ortho.doc for the most current version.

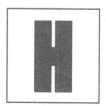

Accredited US Orthopedic Surgery Fellowship Programs

ADULT RECONSTRUCTIVE ORTHOPEDICS

California

Stanford University Program
Program Director: Stuart B. Goodman, MD, PhD
Stanford University
Department of Orthopaedic Surgery
450 Broadway Street, Pavilion C
Redwood City, CA 94063
Tel: (650) 721-7629
Fax: (650) 721-3470
elaus@stanford.edu
http://ortho.stanford.edu

Florida

Jackson Memorial Hospital/Jackson Health System Program
Program Director: Sean P. Scully, MD
University of Miami, Leonard M. Miller School of Medicine
Department of Orthopaedics (D-27)
PO Box 016960
Miami, FL 33101
Tel: (305) 585-1315
Fax: (305) 326-6585
orthoapp@med.miami.edu
www.jhsmiami.org

Illinois

University of Chicago Program
Program Director: Henry A. Finn, MD
University of Chicago, Bone and Joint Replacement Center
Weiss Memorial Hospital
4646 N Marine Drive
Chicago, IL 60640
Tel: (773) 564-5881
Fax: (773) 564-5886
blakinge@surgery.bsd.uchicago.edu
http://www.orthochicago.org

Kentucky

University of Louisville Program
Program Director: Arthur Malkani, MD
University of Louisville School of Medicine
Department of Orthopaedic Surgery
210 East Gray Street, Suite 1003
Louisville, KY 40202
Tel: (502) 852-6902
Fax: (502) 852-7227
cmbing02@gwise.louisville.edu
http://louisville.edu/medschool/orthopaedics

Maryland

Union Memorial Hospital Program
Program Director: Henry R. Boucher,
MD
Union Memorial Hospital
201 East University Parkway
Baltimore, MD 21218
Tel: (410) 554-6755
Fax: (410) 554-2084
meghan.l.shaver@medstar.net
http://www.unionmemorial.org

Michigan

William Beaumont Hospital Program
Program Director: J. Michael Wiater, MD
William Beaumont Hospital
Department of Orthopaedic Surgery
3535 West Thirteen Mile Road, Suite 744
Royal Oak, MI 48073
Tel: (248) 551-3140
Fax: (248) 551-5404
lindsay.cooper@beaumonthospitals.com
https://www.beaumonthospitals.com

Minnesota

*College of Medicine, Mayo Clinic
(Rochester) Program*
Program Director: David G. Lewallen,
MD
Mayo School of Graduate Medical
Education
Siebens 5, 200 First Street SW
Rochester, MN 55905
Tel: (507) 284-3316
Fax: (507) 266-4234
price.natalie@mayo.edu
http://www.mayo.edu

University of Minnesota Program
Program Director: Edward Y. Cheng, MD
University of Minnesota Medical Center
Department of Orthopaedic Surgery
2450 Riverside Avenue South, Suite
R200
Minneapolis, MN 55454
Tel: (612) 273-8043
Fax: (612) 273-8099
wehrw005@umn.edu
http://www.med.umn.edu/ortho

New York

*Albert Einstein College of Medicine at Beth
Israel Medical Center Program*
Program Director: Frances Cuomo, MD
Beth Israel Medical Center
Phillips Ambulatory Care Center
10 Union Square East, Suite 3M
New York, NY 10003
Tel: (212) 844-6938
Fax: (212) 844-6983
fcuomo98@yahoo.com
http://www.einstein.yu.edu

*Hospital for Special Surgery/Cornell
Medical Center Program*
Program Director: Mathias Bostrom,
MD
Hospital for Special Surgery
535 East 70th Street
New York, NY 10021
Tel: (212) 774-2302
Fax: (212) 606-1477
broffmana@hss.edu
http://www.hss.edu/index.htm

Lenox Hill Hospital Program
Program Director: W. Norman Scott,
MD
Lenox Hill Hospital
Department of Orthopedic Surgery
210 East 64th Street
New York, NY 10021
Tel: (212) 434-4340
Fax: (212) 434-4341
klenhardt@iskinstitute.com
http://www.lenoxhillhospital.org

Lenox Hill Hospital Program
Program Director: Jose A. Rodriguez,
MD
Lenox Hill Hospital
William Black Hall, 11th Floor
130 East 77th Street
New York, NY 10075
Tel: (212) 434-4799
Fax: (212) 434-4341
josermd@aol.com
http://www.lenoxhillhospital.org

University at Buffalo Program
Program Director: Kenneth A. Krackow, MD
Buffalo General Hospital
100 High Street, Suite B276
Buffalo, NY 14203
Tel: (716) 859-1256
Fax: (716) 859-4586
comjanet@buffalo.edu
http://www.smbs.buffalo.edu/ortho

North Carolina

Duke University Hospital Program
Program Director: Michael P. Bolognesi, MD
Duke University Medical Center
Division of Orthopaedic Surgery, Box 2923
Durham, NC 27710
Tel: (919) 668-4732
Fax: (919) 681-7795
carolina.manson@duke.edu
http://ortho.surgery.duke.edu

Pennsylvania

Thomas Jefferson University Program
Program Director: William J. Hozack, MD
Thomas Jefferson University
Department of Orthopaedic Surgery
1015 Walnut Street, Room 801 Curtis
Philadelphia, PA 19107
Tel: (215) 955-1500
Fax: (215) 503-0530
susan.randolph@jefferson.edu
http://www.tjuhortho.org

University of Pennsylvania Program
Program Director: Jonathan P. Garino, MD
University of Pennsylvania School of Medicine
39th & Market Streets, 1 Cupp Pavilion
Philadelphia, PA 19104
Tel: (215) 349-8696
Fax: (215) 349-5128
colleen.byrne@uphs.upenn.edu
http://www.uphs.upenn.edu/ortho

University of Pittsburgh Medical Center Medical Education Program
Program Director: Lawrence S. Crossett, MD
University of Pittsburgh School of Medicine
Department of Orthopaedic Surgery
3471 Fifth Avenue
Pittsburgh, PA 15213
Tel: (412) 802-4111
Fax: (412) 802-4120
crossettls@upmc.edu
http://www.orthonet.pitt.edu

Texas

Methodist Hospital (Houston) Program
Program Director: Stephen J. Incavo, MD
The Methodist Hospital (Houston)
6550 Fannin, Suite 2500
Houston, TX 77030
Tel: (713) 441-3892
Fax: (713) 790-6614
jmasterson@tmhs.org
http://www.methodistorthopedics.com

Virginia

University of Virginia Program
Program Director: Khaled J. Saleh, MD, MSc
University of Virginia Health System
PO Box 800159
Charlottesville, VA 22908
Tel: (434) 243-0067
Fax: (434) 243-0242
vmc3y@virginia.edu
http://www.healthsystem.virginia.edu/internet/orthopaedics

Virginia Commonwealth University Health System Program
Program Director: William Jiranek, MD
Virginia Commonwealth University School of Medicine
Department of Orthopaedic Surgery
PO Box 980153
Richmond, VA 23298
Tel: (804) 827-1204
Fax: (804) 827-1728
orthoresprog@vcu.edu
http://www.orthopaedics.vcu.edu

FOOT AND ANKLE ORTHOPEDICS

Alabama

American Sports Medicine Institute Program
Program Director: Angus M. McBryde, MD
American Sports Medicine Institute
2660 10th Avenue South, Suite 505
Birmingham, AL 35205
Tel: (205) 918-2146
Fax: (205) 918-0800
janf@asmi.org
http://www.asmi.org

Arkansas

University of Arkansas for Medical Sciences Program
Program Director: Ruth L. Thomas, MD
University of Arkansas College of Medicine
4301 W Markham, Slot 531
Little Rock, AR 72205
Tel: (501) 686-5673
Fax: (501) 603-1549
thomasruthl@uams.edu
http://www.uams.edu/ortho

Maryland

Mercy Medical Center (Baltimore) Program
Program Director: Mark S. Myerson, MD
Mercy Medical Center, Institute for Foot and Ankle Reconstruction
301 St. Paul Place
Baltimore, MD 21202
Tel: (410) 659-2800
Fax: (410) 659-2999
bcawley@mdmercy.com
http://footandankle.mdmercy.com

Union Memorial Hospital Program
Program Director: Lew C. Schon, MD
Union Memorial Hospital
3333 North Calvert Street, Suite 400
Baltimore, MD 21218
Tel: (410) 554-6865
Fax: (410) 554-2030
patricia.koehler@medstar.net
http://www.unionmemorial.org

New York

Hospital for Special Surgery Program
Program Director: Jonathan Deland, MD
Hospital for Special Surgery
535 East 70th Street
New York, NY 10021
Tel: (212) 606-1655
Fax: (212) 794-4297
academictraining@hss.edu
http://www.hss.edu

University of Rochester Program
Program Director: Benedict DiGiovanni, MD
University of Rochester Medical Center
Department of Orthopaedic Surgery
601 Elmwood Avenue, Box 665
Rochester, NY 14642
Tel: (585) 275-5168
Fax: (585) 756-4721
karen_balta@URMC.Rochester.edu
http://www.urmc.rochester.edu/ortho

North Carolina

Duke University Hospital Program
Program Director: James A. Nunley, MD
Duke University Medical Center
Division of Orthopaedic Surgery, Box 2923
Durham, NC 27710
Tel: (919) 684-4033
Fax: (919) 681-8377
amy.bradley@duke.edu
http://ortho.surgery.duke.edu

Pennsylvania

Penn State University/Milton S. Hershey Medical Center Program
Program Director: Paul J. Juliano, MD
Penn State University/Milton S. Hershey Medical Center
Department of Orthopaedics and Rehabilitation
30 Hope Drive, E.C.089
Hershey, PA 17033
Tel: (717) 531-4833
Fax: (717) 531-0498
orthoresidency@hmc.psu.edu
http://www.pennstatehershey.org

Texas

Baylor University Medical Center Program
Program Director: James W. Brodsky, MD
411 N Washington Avenue, Suite 7000
Dallas, TX 75246
Tel: (214) 823-7090
Fax: (214) 818-1225
http://www.baylorhealth.edu

HAND SURGERY

Alabama

University of Alabama Medical Center Program
Program Director: Thomas R. Hunt, MD
UAB Medical Center
510 20th Street South, FOT 960
Birmingham, AL 35294
Tel: (205) 930-8494
Fax: (205) 930-8569
vicki.allen@ortho.uab.edu
http://www.ortho.uab.edu

Arkansas

University of Arkansas for Medical Sciences Program
Program Director: Robert M. Lumsden, MD
University of Arkansas for Medical Sciences
Department of Orthopaedic Surgery/ Hand Surgery
4301 W Markham, Slot 531
Little Rock, AR 72205
Tel: (501) 686-5595
Fax: (501) 686-7824
dupuylinda@uams.edu
http://www.uams.edu

California

Stanford University Program
Program Director: Amy L. Ladd, MD
Stanford University Medical Center
770 Welch Road, Suite 400
Palo Alto, CA 94304
Tel: (650) 723-6796
Fax: (650) 723-6786
pam.rawls@stanford.edu
http://ortho.stanford.edu

UCLA Medical Center Program
Program Director: Prosper Benhaim, MD
David Geffen School of Medicine at UCLA
10833 Le Conte Avenue, Box 956902, Room 76-143 CHS
Los Angeles, CA 90095
Tel: (310) 206-4468
Fax: (310) 206-0063
pbenhaim@mednet.ucla.edu
http://plasticsurgery.ucla.edu

University of California Davis Health System Program
Program Director: Robert M. Szabo, MD, MPH
UC Davis Medical Center
Department of Orthopaedics
4860 Y Street, Suite 3800
Sacramento, CA 95817
Tel: (916) 734-3678
Fax: (916) 734-7904
barbara.petitt@ucdmc.ucdavis.edu
http://www.ucdmc.ucdavis.edu/ orthopaedics

University of California Irvine/Kaiser Permanente Southern California Program
Program Director: Neil F. Jones, MD
University of California Irvine
101 The City Drive South
Pavilion III, Building 29A
Orange, CA 92868
Tel: (714) 456-5759
Fax: (714) 456-7547
nfjones@uci.edu
http://www.orthopaedicsurgery.uci.edu

University of California San Diego Program
Program Director: Matthew J. Meunier, MD
University of California San Diego Medical Center
200 West Arbor Drive, 8894
San Diego, CA 92103
Tel: (619) 543-5555
Fax: (619) 543-2540
mmeunier@ucsd.edu
http://ortho.ucsd.edu

University of California San Francisco Program
Program Director: Lisa L. Lattanza, MD
University of California, San Francisco, Medical Center
500 Parnassus Avenue, MU-320W
San Francisco, CA 94143
Tel: (415) 476-6043
Fax: (415) 476-1304
lattanza@orthosurg.ucsf.edu
http://orthosurg.ucsf.edu

University of Southern California Medical Center/Los Angeles County Program
Program Director: Stephen B. Schnall, MD
University of Southern California
Division of Plastic & Reconstructive Surgery
1450 San Pablo Street, Suite 2000
Los Angeles, CA 90033
Tel: (323) 226-6931
Fax: (323) 226-6651
ymorgan@usc.edu
http://www.usc.edu/schools/medicine

Colorado

University of Colorado Denver Program
Program Director: Frank A. Scott, MD
University of Colorado School of Medicine
4200 East Ninth Avenue, B-202
Denver, CO 80262
Tel: (303) 724-2961
Fax: (303) 724-2978
patricia.mcfate@uchsc.edu
http://www.uchsc.edu/ortho

Connecticut

University of Connecticut Program
Program Director: H. Kirk Watson, MD
Connecticut Combined Hand Surgery
85 Seymour Street, Suite 816
Hartford, CT 06106
Tel: (860) 251-6773
Fax: (860) 728-3227
hkwatson01@aol.com
http://medicine.uchc.edu

District of Columbia

National Capital Consortium/Walter Reed Program
Program Director: Martin F. Baechler, MD
Walter Reed Army Medical Center
Department of Orthopaedics and Rehabilitation
Orthopedic Surgery Service, 5B25
Washington, DC 20307
Tel: (202) 782-5852
Fax: (202) 782-6845
martin.baechler@us.army.mil
http://www.wramc.amedd.army.mil

Florida

University of Florida Program
Program Director: Paul C. Dell, MD
University of Florida
Orthopaedic & Sports Medicine Institute
PO Box 112727
Gainesville, FL 32611
Tel: (352) 273-7374
Fax: (352) 273-7388
keeneb@ortho.ufl.edu
http://www.ortho.ufl.edu

Jackson Memorial Hospital/Jackson Health System Program
Program Director: Patrick Owens, MD
University of Miami, Leonard M. Miller School of Medicine
Department of Orthopaedics (D-27)
PO Box 016960
Miami, FL 33101
Tel: (305) 326-6000 x4563
Fax: (305) 324-7658
kparis@med.miami.edu
http://www.jhsmiami.org

Illinois

University of Chicago Program
Program Director: Daniel P. Mass, MD
University of Chicago Medical Center
5841 South Maryland Ave, MC 3079
Chicago, IL 60637
Tel: (773) 702-6306
Fax: (773) 702-4378
blakinge@surgery.bsd.uchicago.edu
http://www.orthochicago.org

Indiana

Indiana University School of Medicine Program
Program Director: Jeffrey A. Greenberg, MD, MS
The Indiana Hand Center
8501 Harcourt Road, PO Box 80434
Indianapolis, IN 46280
Tel: (317) 875-9105
Fax: (317) 875-8638
danders@iupui.edu
http://www.orthopaedics.iu.edu

Iowa

University of Iowa Hospitals and Clinics Program
Program Director: Brian D. Adams, MD
University of Iowa Hospitals & Clinics
Orthopaedic Surgery
200 Hawkins Dr, 01008 JPP
Iowa City, IA 52242
Tel: (319) 353-6222
Fax: (319) 353-6754
karissa-ockander@uiowa.edu
http://www.uihealthcare.com

Maryland

Union Memorial Hospital Program
Program Director: Thomas J. Graham, MD
Union Memorial Hospital
The Curtis National Hand Center
3333 North Calvert Street
Baltimore, MD 21218
Tel: (410) 554-6593
Fax: (410) 554-4363
tori.wilson@medstar.net
http://www.unionmemorial.org

Massachusetts

Beth Israel Deaconess Medical Center/ Harvard Medical School Program
Program Director: Joseph Upton, MD
Beth Israel Deaconess Medical Center
Department of Orthopaedic Surgery
330 Brookline Avenue, Stoneman 10th Floor
Boston, MA 02215
Tel: (617) 667-3758

Fax: (617) 667-9122
gbrahmer@bidmc.harvard.edu
http://www.bidmc.org

Brigham and Women's Hospital/Harvard Medical School Program
Program Director: Barry P. Simmons, MD
Brigham and Women's Hospital
Department of Orthopedic Surgery
75 Francis Street
Boston, MA 02115
Tel: (617) 732-8550
Fax: (617) 732-6397
dsheehan@partners.org
http://www.brighamandwomens.org

Massachusetts General Hospital/Harvard Medical School Program
Program Director: Chaitanya S. Mudgal, MD, MS
Massachusetts General Hospital
Department of Orthopaedic Surgery
Yawkey Building, Suite 3C
55 Fruit Street
Boston, MA 02114
Tel: (617) 643-0149
Fax: (617) 724-8532
chilgendorf@partners.org
http://www.massgeneral.org

Tufts Medical Center Program
Program Director: Charles Cassidy, MD
Tufts Medical Center
Department of Orthopaedics, Box 26
800 Washington Street
Boston, MA 02111
Tel: (617) 636-5172
Fax: (617) 636-5178
jdolph@tuftsmedicalcenter.org
http://www.tuftsmedicalcenter.org

University of Massachusetts Program
Program Director: Marci Jones, MD
University of Massachusetts
Department of Orthopedics, H4-529
55 Lake Avenue North
Worcester, MA 01655
Tel: (508) 856-4262
Fax: (508) 334-5151
michelle.auger@umassmed.edu
http://www.umassmed.edu/orthopedics

Minnesota

*College of Medicine, Mayo Clinic
(Rochester) Program*
Program Director: Richard A. Berger,
MD, Ph.D
Mayo School of Graduate Medical
Education
200 First Street, SW
Rochester, MN 55905
Tel: (507) 284-3316
Fax: (507) 266-2533
price.natalie@mayo.edu
http://www.mayo.edu/msgme/ortho-
surg-programs.html

University of Minnesota Program
Program Director: Matthew D. Putnam,
MD
University of Minnesota
Department of Orthopaedic Surgery
2450 Riverside Avenue South, Suite
R200
Minneapolis, MN 55454
Tel: (651) 273-1177
Fax: (651) 273-8099
olson073@umn.edu
http://www.med.umn.edu/ortho

Mississippi

*University of Mississippi Medical Center
Program*
Program Director: William B. Geissler,
MD
University of Mississippi Medical Center
2500 North State Street
Jackson, MS 39216
Tel: (601) 984-5153
Fax: (601) 984-5151
salexander@orthopedics.umsmed.edu
http://gme.umc.edu

Missouri

*Washington University/Barnes-Jewish
Hospital/Saint Louis Children's
Hospital Consortium Program*
Program Director: Martin I. Boyer, MD
Washington University School of
Medicine
Department of Orthopedic Surgery

660 South Euclid Avenue, Campus Box
8233
St. Louis, MO 63110
Tel: (314) 747-4705
Fax: (314) 747-2643
addisonk@wudosis.wustl.edu
http://medschool.wustl.edu

New Jersey

*UMDNJ-New Jersey Medical School
Program*
Program Director: Virak Tan, MD
UMDNJ-NJMS, North Jersey
Orthopedic Institute
Department of Orthopaedics
90 Bergen Street, DOC 7300
PO Box 1709
Newark, NJ 07101
Tel: (973) 972-0763
Fax: (973) 972-1080
birthwma@umdnj.edu
http://njms.umdnj.edu

New Mexico

University of New Mexico Program
Program Director: Moheb S. Moneim,
MD
University of New Mexico
Department of Orthopaedics and
Rehabilitation
MSC10 5600
1 University of New Mexico
Albuquerque, NM 87131
Tel: (505) 272-6472
Fax: (505) 272-8098
jroberts@salud.unm.edu
http://hsc.unm.edu/som

New York

*Albert Einstein College of Medicine at Beth
Israel Medical Center Program*
Program Director: Charles P. Melone, MD
Beth Israel Medical Center
321 East 34th Street
New York, NY 10016
Tel: (212) 340-0000
Fax: (212) 340-0035
admissions@aecom.yu.edu
http://www.einstein.yu.edu

*Columbia University/New York
Presbyterian Hospital Program*
Program Director: Melvin P.
Rosenwasser, MD
Columbia University Medical Center
622 West 168th Street, PH11-Center
New York, NY 10032
Tel: (212) 305-8036
Fax: (212) 305-6193
finnole@nyp.org
http://www.columbiaortho.org

*Hospital for Special Surgery/Cornell
Medical Center Program*
Program Director: Scott W. Wolfe, MD
Hospital for Special Surgery
535 East 70th Street
New York, NY 10021
Tel: (212) 606-1466
Fax: (212) 606-1477
academictraining@hss.edu
http://www.hss.edu

Mount Sinai School of Medicine Program
Program Director: Michael Hausman,
MD
Mount Sinai School of Medicine
5 East 98th Street, Box 1188
New York, NY 10029
Tel: (212) 241-1621
Fax: (212) 241-9429
amanda.mercado@mountsinai.org
http://www.mountsinai.org

*New York University School of Medicine/
Hospital for Joint Diseases Program*
Program Director: Martin A. Posner, MD
NYUMC Hospital for Joint Diseases
301 East 17th Street, Room 1402
New York, NY 10003
Tel: (212) 598-6509
Fax: (212) 369-4742
randie.godette@nyumc.org
http://www.med.nyu.edu/orthosurgery

*Saint Luke's-Roosevelt Hospital Center
Program*
Program Director: Steven Z. Glickel, MD
Saint Luke's-Roosevelt Hospital Center
1000 Tenth Avenue
New York, NY 10019

Tel: (212) 523-7590
Fax: (212) 523-7592
sglickel@msn.com
http://www.slrhc.org

SUNY at Stony Brook Program
Program Director: Lawrence Hurst, MD
Stony Brook University Hospital
Department of Orthopaedics
HSC T18-089
Stony Brook, NY 11794
Tel: (631) 444-1487
Fax: (631) 444-3502
gayle.siegel@sunysb.edu
http://www.hsc.stonybrook.edu/som/
orthopaedic/residency

SUNY Upstate Medical University Program
Program Director: Brian J. Harley, MD
SUNY Upstate Medical University
Department of Orthopedic Surgery
750 East Adams Street
Syracuse, NY 13210
Tel: (315) 464-5226
Fax: (315) 464-6470
bordeauj@upstate.edu
http://www.upstate.edu/ortho

University at Buffalo Program
Program Director: Owen J. Moy, MD
Hand and Shoulder Center of Western
NY
Kaleida Health-Millard Fillmore Gates
Hospital
3 Gates Circle
Buffalo, NY 14209
Tel: (716) 887-4040
Fax: (716) 887-5090
info@buffalohands.com
http://www.buffalohandandshoulder.com

University of Rochester Program
Program Director: Richard J. Miller, MD
University of Rochester Medical Center
Department of Orthopaedics
601 Elmwood Avenue, Box 665
Rochester, NY 14642
Tel: (585) 275-5168
Fax: (585) 756-4721
karen_balta@urmc.rochester.edu
http://www.urmc.rochester.edu/ortho

North Carolina

Duke University Hospital Program
Program Director: David S. Ruch, MD
Duke University Medical Center
Division of Orthopaedic Surgery, Box
  2923
Durham, NC 27710
Tel: (919) 684-3170
Fax: (919) 681-7672
wendy.thompson@duke.edu
http://ortho.surgery.duke.edu

*Wake Forest University School of Medicine
  Program*
Program Director: L. Andrew Koman,
  MD
Wake Forest University School of
  Medicine
Department of Orthopaedic Surgery
Medical Center Boulevard, #1070
Winston-Salem, NC 27517
Tel: (336) 716-3946
Fax: (336) 716-3861
hermance@wfubmc.edu
http://www.wfubmc.edu

Ohio

Cleveland Clinic Foundation Program
Program Director: Peter J. Evans, MD,
  PhD
The Cleveland Clinic Foundation
Department of Orthopaedic Surgery/A50
9500 Euclid Avenue
Cleveland, OH 44195
Tel: (216) 444-0332
Fax: (216) 445-3694
paciorl@ccf.org
http://my.clevelandclinic.org/ortho

*University of Cincinnati/Mary S. Stern
  Foundation/University Hospital
  Program*
Program Director: Peter J. Stern, MD
The Mary S. Stern Foundation
538 Oak Street, Suite 200
Cincinnati, OH 45219
Tel: (513) 961-4360
Fax: (513) 961-7742
robbie.cornelison@healthall.com
http://www.handsurg.com

Oklahoma

Integris Baptist Medical Center Program
Program Director: Ghazi M. Rayan, MD
Integris Baptist Medical Center
Graduate Medical Education
3300 NW Expressway, #700
Oklahoma City, OK 73112
Tel: (405) 552-0926
Fax: (405) 552-5102
annette.kezbers@integrisok.com
http://www.integris-health.com/
    INTEGRIS/en-US/Locations/okc-
    North/BMC-okc

Pennsylvania

Allegheny General Hospital Program
Program Director: Mark E. Baratz, MD
Allegheny General Hospital
1307 Federal Street, 2nd floor
Pittsburgh, PA 15212
Tel: (412) 359-6501
Fax: (412) 359-6265
polzak@wpahs.org
http://www.wpahs.org/agh

Hamot Medical Center Program
Program Director: John D. Lubahn, MD
Hamot Medical Center
201 State Street
Erie, PA 16550
Tel: (814) 877-6257
Fax: (814) 877-4010
pat.rogers@hamot.org
http://www.hamot.org

Thomas Jefferson University Program
Program Director: A. Lee Osterman, MD
The Philadelphia Hand Center
834 Chestnut Street, Suite G114
Philadelphia, PA 19107
Tel: (215) 629-0980
Fax: (610) 768-4469
susan.randolph@jefferson.edu
http://www.tjuhortho.org

University of Pennsylvania Program
Program Director: David R. Steinberg,
  MD
Hospital of the University of Pennsylvania
Department of Orthopaedic Surgery

3400 Spruce Street, 2 Silverstein
Philadelphia, PA 19104
Tel: (215) 662-3957
Fax: (215) 615-4111
barbara.weinraub@uphs.upenn.edu
http://www.uphs.upenn.edu/ortho/aca-
demics

*University of Pittsburgh Medical Center
Medical Education Program*
Program Director: Joseph E. Imbriglia,
MD
University Health Center of Pittsburgh
6001 Stonewood Drive, 2nd Floor
Wexford, PA 15090
Tel: (724) 933-3850 x168
Fax: (724) 933-3861
dbuyna@handupperex.com
http://www.orthonet.pitt.edu

Rhode Island

Brown University Program
Program Director: Edward Akelman,
MD
Rhode Island Hospital
2 Dudley Street, Suite 200
Providence, RI 02905
Tel: (401) 457-1512
Fax: (401) 831-5874
brownuhandfel@yahoo.com
http://biomed.brown.edu/orthopaedics

Tennessee

Vanderbilt University Program
Program Director: Donald H. Lee, MD
Vanderbilt Orthopaedic Institute
Medical Center East
1215 21st Avenue South
South Tower, Suite 4200
Nashville, TN 37232
Tel: (615) 322-4683
Fax: (615) 343-8989
karen.shelton@vanderbilt.edu
http://www.vanderbilthealth.com/
orthopaedics

Texas

Baylor College of Medicine Program
Program Director: Michael J. Epstein,
MD

Baylor College of Medicine
Department of Orthopedic Surgery
1709 Dryden Road, 12th Floor
Houston, TX 77030
Tel: (713) 986-5840
Fax: (713) 986-5841
ortho@bcm.edu
http://www.bcm.edu/ortho

*University of Texas Health Science Center
at San Antonio Program*
Program Director: William C. Pederson,
MD
The University of Texas Health Science
Center at San Antonio
Department of Orthopaedics
7703 Floyd Curl Drive - MC 7774
San Antonio TX 78229
Tel: (210) 558-7025
Fax: (210) 558-4664
carlawaller@yahoo.com
http://www.uthscsa.edu/orthopaedics

Utah

University of Utah Program
Program Director: Douglas T.
Hutchinson, MD
University of Utah Medical Center
590 Wakara Way
Salt Lake City, UT 84108
Tel: (801) 587-5448
Fax: (801) 587-5411
elise.collins@hsc.utah.edu
http://medicine.utah.edu/orthopaedics

Washington

University of Washington Program
Program Director: Thomas E. Trumble,
MD
University of Washington School of
Medicine
Department of Orthopedics and Sports
Medicine
4245 Roosevelt Way NE, Box 354740
Seattle, WA 98105
Tel: (206) 598-1879
Fax: (206) 598-9979
uwhand@u.washington.edu
http://www.orthop.washington.edu

Wisconsin

Medical College of Wisconsin Affiliated Hospitals Program
Program Director: Roger A. Daley, MD, PhD
Medical College of Wisconsin
Department of Plastic Surgery
8700 Watertown Plank Road
Milwaukee, WI 53226
Tel: (414) 805-5465
Fax: (414) 805-7499
bruening@mcw.edu
http://www.mcw.edu/orthopaedicsurgery.htm

MUSCULOSKELETAL ONCOLOGY

District of Columbia

Washington Hospital Center/Georgetown University Program
Program Director: Robert M. Henshaw, MD
Washington Hospital Center
110 Irving Street, NW, Suite C2173
Washington, DC 20010
Tel: (202) 877-3970
Fax: (202) 877-8959
ortho@mhg.edu
http://www.whcenter.org

Florida

Jackson Memorial Hospital/Jackson Health System Program
Program Director: H. Thomas Temple, MD
University of Miami, Leonard M. Miller School of Medicine
Department of Orthopaedics (D-27)
PO Box 016960
Miami, FL 33101
Tel: (305) 585-1315
Fax: (305) 324-7658
orthoapp@med.miami.edu
www.jhsmiami.org

University of Florida Program
Program Director: Mark T. Scarborough, MD
University of Florida, Orthopaedics and Sports Medicine Institute
PO Box 112727
Gainesville, FL 32611
Tel: (352) 273-7365
Fax: (352) 273-7388
gallaks@ortho.ufl.edu
http://www.ortho.ufl.edu

Illinois

University of Chicago Program
Program Director: Terrance Peabody, MD
University of Chicago Medical Center
5841 South Maryland Avenue, MC 3079
Chicago, IL 60637
Tel: (773) 702-3442
Fax: (773) 702-4384
tpeabody@surgery.bsd.uchicago.edu
http://www.uchospitals.edu

Massachusetts

Massachusetts General Hospital/Harvard Medical School Program
Program Director: Francis J. Hornicek, MD, PhD
Massachusetts General Hospital
55 Fruit Street
Yawkey 3700
Boston, MA 02114
Tel: (617) 726-8731
Fax: (617) 726-6823
dsheehan@partners.org
http://www.massgeneral.org

Minnesota

College of Medicine, Mayo Clinic (Rochester) Program
Program Director: Michael G. Rock, MD
Mayo School of Graduate Medical Education
Siebens 5, 200 First Street SW
Rochester, MN 55905
Tel: (507) 284-3316
Fax: (507) 266-4234
price.natalie@mayo.edu
http://www.mayo.edu

New Jersey

UMDNJ-New Jersey Medical School Program
Program Director: Joseph Benevenia, MD
UMDNJ-NJMS, North Jersey
    Orthopaedic Institute
Department of Orthopaedics
90 Bergen Street, DOC Suite 7300
Newark, NJ 07101
Tel: (973) 972-2153
Fax: (973) 972-1080
birthwma@umdnj.edu
http://njms.umdnj.edu/departments/
    orthopaedics

New York

Memorial Sloan-Kettering Cancer Center Program
Program Director: John Healey, MD
Memorial Sloan-Kettering Cancer Center
1275 York Avenue
New York, NY 10065
Tel: (212) 639-7610
Fax: (212) 717-3573
okeefek@mskcc.org
http://www.mskcc.org/mskcc/html/44.
    cfm

Tennessee

Vanderbilt University Program
Program Director: Ginger E. Holt, MD
Vanderbilt Orthopaedic Institute
Medical Center East
1215 21st Avenue South
South Tower, Suite 4200
Nashville, TN 37232
Tel: (615) 343-0825
Fax: (615) 322-7556
marla.johnson@vanderbilt.edu
http://www.vanderbilthealth.com/
    orthopaedics

Texas

University of Texas M.D. Anderson Cancer Center Program
Program Director: Valerae O. Lewis, BS, MD
The University of Texas M.D. Anderson
    Cancer Center

Department of Orthopaedic Oncology
1400 Holcome Boulevard
PO Box 301402, Unit 408
Houston, TX 77030
Tel: (713) 745-4568
Fax: (713) 792-8448
mdmartin@mdanderson.org
http://www.mdanderson.org

ORTHOPEDIC SPORTS MEDICINE

Alabama

American Sports Medicine Institute Program
Program Director: James Andrews, MD
American Sports Medicine Institute
2660 10th Avenue South, Suite 505
Birmingham, AL 35205
Tel: (205) 918-2146
Fax: (205) 918-0800
janf@asmi.org
http://www.asmi.org

University of South Alabama Program
Program Director: Albert W. Pearsall, MD
University of South Alabama
Department of Orthopaedic Surgery
3421 Medical Park Drive, Building #2
Mobile, AL 36693
Tel: (251) 665-8250
Fax: (251) 665-8565
gdriver@usouthal.edu
http://www.southalabama.edu/com/ortho

Arizona

University of Arizona Program
Program Director: William A. Grana, MD, MPH
University of Arizona Health Sciences
    Center
Department of Orthopaedic Surgery
PO Box 245064
Tucson, AZ 85724
Tel: (520) 626-9245
Fax: (520) 626-2668
sbrandes@emedicine.arizona.edu
http://www.bones.arizona.edu

California

Congress Medical Associates Program
Program Director: Gregory J. Adamson, MD
Congress Medical Associates
800 South Raymond Ave, 2nd Floor
Pasadena, CA 91105
Tel: (626) 795-8051
Fax: (626) 795-0356
http://www.congressmedical.com

Kaiser Permanente Southern California (Orange County) Program
Program Director: Brent R. Davis, MD
Sand Canyon Medical Office and Surgery Center
Department of Orthopaedic Surgery
6670 Alton Parkway
Irvine, CA 92618
Tel: (949) 932-5002
brent.r.davis@kp.org
http://residency.kp.org/scal

Kaiser Permanente Southern California (San Diego) Program
Program Director: Donald C. Fithian, MD
Kaiser Permanente Southern California
250 Travelodge Drive
El Cajon, CA 92020
Tel: (619) 441-3142
Fax: (619) 441-3136
marcia.m.griffith@kp.org
http://residency.kp.org/scal

Kerlan-Jobe Orthopedic Clinic Program
Program Director: Neal S. ElAttrache, MD
Kerlan-Jobe Orthopaedic Clinic
6801 Park Terrace, Suite 500
Los Angeles, CA 90045
Tel: (310) 665-7257
Fax: (310) 665-7145
kjofresearch@aol.com
http://www.kerlanjobe.com

Long Beach Memorial Medical Center Program
Program Director: Peter R. Kurzweil, MD
Long Beach Memorial Medical Center
2801 Atlantic Avenue, PO Box 1428
Long Beach, CA 90806
Tel: (562) 933-3800
Fax: (562) 933-3888
bbryant@memorialcare.org
http://www.memorialcare.org

San Diego Arthroscopy and Sports Medicine Program
Program Director: James P. Tasto, MD
San Diego Sports Medicine and Orthopaedic Center
6719 Alvarado Road, Suite 200
San Diego, CA 92120
Tel: (619) 225-5018
Fax: (619) 229-5011
http://www.sdsm.net

Santa Monica Orthopedic and Sports Medicine Group Program
Program Director: Bert Mandelbaum, MD
Santa Monica Orthopaedic and Sports Medicine Group
2020 Santa Monica Boulevard, Suite 400
Santa Monica, CA 90404
Tel: (310) 829-2663
Fax: (310) 315-0326
dianew@smog-ortho.net
http://www.smogshoulder.com

Southern California Orthopedic Institute Program
Program Director: Richard D. Ferkel, MD
Southern California Orthopedic Institute
6815 Noble Street
Van Nuys, CA 91405
Tel: (818) 901-6600 x1526
Fax: (818) 901-6660
eobrien@scoi.com
http://www.scoi.com

Sports Clinic (Laguna Hills) Program
Program Director: Wesley M. Nottage,
MD
The Sports Clinic Orthopaedic Medical
Associates, Inc.
23961 Calle de la Magdalena #229
Laguna Hills, CA 92653
Tel: (949) 581-7001
Fax: (949) 581-8410
bigdog492653@yahoo.com
http://www.thesportsclinic.net

Stanford University Program
Program Director: Marc R. Safran, MD
Stanford University
Department of Orthopaedic Surgery
450 Broadway Street, Pavilion C, 4th
Floor
Redwood City, CA 94063
Tel: (650) 721-7618
Fax: (650) 721-3470
jackieg@stanford.edu
http://ortho.stanford.edu

University of California (San Francisco)
Program
Program Director: Christina R. Allen,
MD
University of California, San Francisco
Department of Sports Medicine
500 Parnassus Avenue, MU-320W
San Francisco, CA 94143
Tel: (415) 476-6043
Fax: (415) 476-1304
sportsfellow@orthosurg.ucsf.edu
http://www.ucsfhealth.org

University of Southern California
Orthopaedic Surgery Associates
Program
Program Director: James E. Tibone, MD
University of Southern California
Department of Orthopaedic Surgery
1200 North State Street, GNH 3900
Los Angeles, CA 90033
Tel: (323) 442-5868
Fax: (323) 226-4051
tyranny@usc.edu
http://www.usc.edu/schools/medicine

UCLA Medical Center Program
Program Director: David McAllister, MD
David Geffen School of Medicine at
UCLA
10833 Le Conte Avenue, Room 76-
143CHS
Los Angeles, CA 90095
Tel: (310) 825-6557
Fax: (310) 825-1311
orthoeducation@mednet.ucla.edu
http://ortho.ucla.edu/

Colorado

Aspen Sports Medicine Foundation Program
Program Director: Norman L. Harris,
MD
Orthopedic Associates of Aspen &
Glenwood/AFSMER
100 E Main Street, Suite 101
Aspen, CO 81611
Tel: (970) 920-4151
Fax: (970) 544-1777
asmf@orthop.com
http://www.orthop.com

Panorama Orthopedics & Spine Center
Program
Program Director: James Johnson, MD,
MPH
Panorama Orthopedics & Spine Center
660 Golden Ridge Road, Suite 250
Golden, CO 80401
Tel: (303) 233-1223
Fax: (303) 233-8755
jjohnson@panoramaortho.com
http://www.panoramaortho.com

Steadman Hawkins Clinic (Denver)
Program
Program Director: Theodore F. Schlegel,
MD
Steadman Hawkins Clinic - Denver
8200 E Belleview Avenue, Suite 615
Greenwood Village, CO 80111
Tel: (303) 694-3333
Fax: (303) 694-9666
therbert@shcdenver.com
http://www.shcdenver.com/Home/
tabid/9435/Default.aspx

Steadman Hawkins Clinic Program
Program Director: J. Richard Steadman, MD
Steadman Hawkins Clinic
181 West Meadow Drive, Suite 400
Vail, CO 81657
Tel: (970) 479-5782
Fax: (970) 479-5835
keepck@steadman-hawkins.com
http://www.steadman-hawkins.com

University of Colorado Denver Program
Program Director: Eric McCarty, MD
University of Colorado
Department of Orthopaedics
311 Mapleton Avenue
Boulder, CO 80304
Tel: (303) 441-2219
Fax: (303) 441-2230
patricia.mcfate@uchsc.edu
http://www.uchsc.edu/ortho

Connecticut

University of Connecticut Program
Program Director: Robert A. Arciero, M.D.
New England Musculoskeletal Institute
Medical Arts & Research Building
University of Connecticut Health Center
263 Farmington Avenue
Farmington, CT 06030
Tel: (860) 679-6645
Fax: (860) 679-6649
tolisano@nso.uchc.edu
http://connecticutmusculoskeletalinstitute.com

Florida

Andrews/Paulos Research and Education Institute Program
Program Director: Lonnie E. Paulos, MD
Andrews Institute for Orthopaedics & Sports Medicine
1040 Gulf Breeze Parkway
Gulf Breeze, FL 32561
Tel: (850) 916-8583
Fax: (850) 916-3710
sherry.gammache@theandrewsinstitute.com
http://www.andrewsortho.com

Harlan Selesnick, MD/Doctors Hospital Program
Program Director: Harlan Selesnick, MD
HealthSouth Medical Office Building
1150 Campo Sano Avenue, Suite 301
Coral Gables, FL 33146
Tel: (786) 308-3350
Fax: (786) 308-3379
info@sportsmedicinemiami.com
http://www.sportsmedicinemiami.com

UHZ Sports Medicine/Doctors Hospital Fellowship
Program Director: John W. Uribe, MD
UHZ Sports Medicine Institute
1150 Campo Sano Avenue, Suite 200
Coral Gables, FL 33146
Tel: (305) 669-3320
Fax: (786) 268-6279
norad@baptisthealth.net
http://www.uhzsmi.com

University of South Florida Program
Program Director: David Leffers, MD
University of South Florida
Department of Orthopaedics and Sports Medicine
3500 E. Fletcher Avenue, Suite 511, MDC106
Tampa, FL 33613
Tel: (813) 396-9639
Fax: (813) 396-9195
ajoyce@health.usf.edu
http://health.usf.edu/nocms/medicine/orthopaedic

Georgia

Atlanta Sports Medicine Foundation Program
Program Director: Scott D. Gillogly, MD
Atlanta Sports Medicine & Orthopaedic Center
3200 Downwood Circle NW, Suite 500
Atlanta, GA 30327
Tel: (404) 352-4500 x649
Fax: (404) 693-9003
drheault@atlantasportsmedicine.com
http://www.atlantasportsmedicine.com

Emory University Program
Program Director: Spero G. Karas, MD
Emory University
Department of Orthopaedics
59 Executive Park Drive South, Suite 1000
Atlanta, GA 30329
Tel: (404) 778-7204
Fax: (404) 727-5456
kstrozi@emory.edu
http://www.orthopaedics.emory.edu

Hughston Foundation Program
Program Director: Champ L. Baker, MD
Hughston Foundation, Inc.
6262 Veteran's Parkway
PO Box 9517
Columbus, GA 31908
Tel: (706) 494-3365
Fax: (706) 494-3379
froberts@hughston.com
http://www.hughstonfoundation.com

Illinois

Rush University Medical Center Program
Program Director: Bernard R. Bach, MD
Rush University
Department of Orthopedic Surgery
1653 W. Congress Parkway, 1471 Jelke
Chicago, IL 60612
Tel: (312) 942-4301
Fax: (312) 942-2101
phyllis_j_velez@rush.edu
http://www.rush.edu/professionals/gme

University of Chicago Program
Program Director: Sherwin S. Ho, MD, BA
University of Chicago Medical Center
5841 South Maryland Ave, MC 3079
Chicago, IL 60637-3079
Tel: (773) 702-5978
Fax: (773) 702-0554
sho@surgery.bsd.uchicago.edu
http://surgery.uchicago.edu/specialties/orthopaedic

University of Illinois College of Medicine at Chicago Program
Program Director: Preston M. Wolin, MD

University of Illinois Medical Center
Center for Athletic Medicine
830 West Diversey, Suite 300
Chicago, IL 60614
Tel: (773) 248-4150
Fax: (773) 248-4291
pwolin@athleticmed.com
http://www.chicago.medicine.uic.edu

Indiana

Indiana University School of Medicine/ Methodist Sports Medicine Program
Program Director: Arthur C. Rettig, MD
Methodist Sports Medicine Center
201 North Pennsylvania Parkway, Suite 325
Indianapolis, IN 46280
Tel: (317) 817-1227
Fax: (317) 817-1220
phunker@methodistsports.com
http://www.methodistsports.com

Iowa

University of Iowa Hospitals and Clinics Program
Program Director: Brian Wolf, MD, MS
University of Iowa
Department of Orthopaedics and Rehabilitation
2701 Prairie Meadow Drive
Iowa City, IA 52242
Tel: (319) 353-7954
Fax: (319) 384-9306
brian-wolf@uiowa.edu
http://www.uihealthcare.com/depts/med/orthopaedicsurgery

Kansas

University of Missouri at Kansas City Program
Program Director: Jon E. Browne, MD
University of Missouri at Kansas City
3651 College Boulevard, Suite 100A
Leawood, KS 66211
Tel: (913) 319-7546
Fax: (913) 319-7691
maryz@osmckc.com
http://www.med.umkc.edu

Kentucky

University of Kentucky College of Medicine Program
Program Director: Robert Hosey, MD
University of Kentucky Sports Medicine Center
K302 Kentucky Clinic
Lexington, KY 40536-0284
Tel: (859) 323-6712
Fax: (859) 323-2412
jthoma2@email.uky.edu
http://www.mc.uky.edu/familymedicine

Louisiana

Ochsner Clinic Foundation Program
Program Director: Deryk G. Jones, MD
Ochsner Clinic Foundation
1514 Jefferson Highway
New Orleans, LA 70121
Tel: (504) 842-6793
Fax: (504) 736-4810
gchaisson@ochsner.org
http://www.ochsner.org

Maryland

Union Memorial Hospital Program
Program Director: Leslie Matthews, MD
Union Memorial Hospital
3333 N. Calvert Street, Suite 400
Baltimore, MD 21218
Tel: (410) 554-6865
Fax: (410) 261-8105
patricia.koehler@medstar.net
http://www.unionmemorial.org

Massachusetts

Boston University Medical Center Program
Program Director: Anthony A. Schepsis, MD
Boston University Medical Center
715 Albany Street, DOB-808
Boston, MA 02118
Tel: (617) 638-8934
Fax: (617)6 38-8493
lynnette.stlouis@bmc.org
http://www.bumc.bu.edu/orthopaedics

Children's Hospital Boston Program
Program Director: Lyle J. Micheli, MD
Children's Hospital Boston
Division of Sports Medicine
319 Longwood Avenue
Boston, MA 02115
Tel: (617) 355-6247
Fax: (617) 730-0694
maria.maginnis@childrens.harvard.edu
http://www.childrenshospital.org

Massachusetts General Hospital/Harvard Medical School Program
Program Director: Thomas Gill, MD
Massachusetts General Hospital
175 Cambridge Street
Suite 400, Sports Medicine
Boston, MA 02114
Tel: (617) 726-7500
Fax: (617) 643-2030
tgill@partners.org
http://www2.massgeneral.org/sports

New England Baptist Hospital Program
Program Director: Mark E. Steiner, MD
New England Baptist Hospital
Department of Orthopedics
125 Parker Hill Avenue
Boston, MA 02120
Tel: (617) 754-5413
Fax: (617) 754-6443
msteiner@caregroup.harvard.edu
http://www.nebh.org

University of Massachusetts Program
Program Director: Brian D. Busconi, MD
University of Massachusetts, Worchester
Department of Orthopedics and Physical Rehabilitation
55 Lake Avenue North
Worcester, MA 01655
Tel: (508) 856-4262
Fax: (508) 334-7273
michelle.auger@umassmed.edu
http://www.umassmed.edu/orthopedics

Michigan

Detroit Medical Center Program
Program Director: Stephen Lemos, MD, PhD
Detroit Medical Center
28800 Ryan Road, Suite 120
Warren, MI 48092
Tel: (586) 558-2867
Fax: (586) 558-4651
lgross@dmc.org
http://www.dmcsurgeryhospital.org

University of Michigan Program
Program Director: Robert B. Kiningham, MD, MA, FACSM
University of Michigan
Department of Family Medicine
L2003 Women's Hospital
1500 E. Medical Center Drive
Ann Arbor, MI 48109-5239
Tel: (734) 232-6776
Fax: (734) 615-2687
rkiningh@med.umich.edu
http://www.med.umich.edu

Wayne State University/Detroit Medical Center Program
Program Director: Robert A. Teitge, MD
Wayne State University
Department of Orthopaedic Surgery
18100 Oakwood Boulevard, Suite 300
Dearborn, MI 48124
Tel: (313) 745-3456
Fax: (313) 966-0880
dmitchel4@dmc.org
http://www.dmc.org

William Beaumont Hospital Program
Program Director: Kyle Anderson, MD
William Beaumont Hospital
3535 West 13 Mile Road, Suite 744
Royal Oak, MI 48073
Tel: (248) 551-0426
Fax: (248) 551-5404
lindsay.cooper@beaumonthospitals.com
www.beaumonthospitals.com/gme

Henry Ford Hospital Program
Program Director: Henry Goitz, MD
Henry Ford Hospital
Center for Athletic Medicine
3525 Second Avenue
Detroit, MI 48202
Tel: (313) 972-4076
Fax: (313) 942-4202
hgoitz1@hfhs.org
http://www.henryford.com

Minnesota

Fairview Sports and Orthopedic Care Program
Program Director: J. P. Smith, MD
Fairview Sports and Orthopedic Care
Pondview Medical Building
501 Nicollet Boulevard, #100
Burnsville, MN 55337
Tel: (612) 273-9196
Fax: (612) 273-4560
lhenn1@fairview.org
http://www.fairview.org

The Orthopaedic Center Program
Program Director: David A. Fischer, MD
TRIA Orthopaedic Center
8100 Northland Drive
Bloomington, MN 55431
Tel: (952) 831-8326
Fax: (952) 831-1626
d.fischermn@comcast.net
http://www.tria.com

Mississippi

Mississippi Sports Medicine & Orthopaedic Center Program
Program Director: Larry D. Field, MD
Mississippi Sports Medicine & Orthopaedic Center
1325 East Fortification Street
Jackson, MS 39202
Tel: (601) 354-4488
Fax: (601) 914-1835
lrhodes@msmoc.com
http://www.msmoc.com

Missouri

Washington University/Barnes-Jewish Hospital/Saint Louis Children's Hospital Consortium Program
Program Director: Matthew J. Matava, MD
Washington University
Department of Orthopedic Surgery
660 South Euclid Avenue, Campus Box 8233
St. Louis, MO 63110
Tel: (314) 514-3569
Fax: (314) 514-3689
haegeleb@wudosis.wustl.edu
http://www.ortho.wustl.edu

New Mexico

New Mexico Orthopaedics Program
Program Director: Anthony F. Pachelli, MD
New Mexico Orthopaedics Fellowship Foundation
201 Cedar SE, Suite 6600
Albuquerque, NM 87106
Tel: (505) 724-3236
Fax: (505) 742-4384
nmfellowship@nmortho.net
http://nmorthosportsfellow.com

Taos Orthopaedic Institute and Research Foundation Program
Program Director: James H. Lubowitz, MD
Taos Orthopaedic Institute
1219-A Gusdorf Road
Taos, NM 87571
Tel: (575) 758-0009
Fax: (575) 758-8736
info@taosortho.com
http://www.taosortho.com

University of New Mexico Program
Program Director: Daniel Wascher, MD
University of New Mexico School of Medicine
Department of Orthopaedics, MSC10 5600
1 University of New Mexico
Albuquerque, NM 87131

Tel: (505) 272-6472
Fax: (505) 272-8098
jroberts@salud.unm.edu
http://hsc.unm.edu/som

New York

Hospital for Special Surgery/Cornell Medical Center Program
Program Director: Scott Rodeo, MD
Hospital for Special Surgery
535 East 70th Street
New York, NY 10021
Tel: (212) 606-1513
Fax: (212) 774-2414
academictraining@hss.edu
http://www.hss.edu/index.htm

Keller Army Community Hospital Program
Program Director: Steven J. Svoboda, MD
Keller Army Community Hospital
Orthopaedic Service
900 Washington Road
West Point, NY 10996
Tel: (845) 938-6620
Fax: (845) 938-6806
steven.svoboda@amedd.army.mil
http://kach.amedd.army.mil

Lenox Hill Hospital Program
Program Director: Barton Nisonson, MD
Lenox Hill Hospital
130 East 77th Street, 11th Floor
New York, NY 10075
Tel: (212) 570-9120
Fax: (212) 434-4341
orthopedics@mindspring.com
http://www.lenoxhillhospital.org

New York Presbyterian Hospital (Columbia Campus) Program
Program Director: Louis U. Bigliani, MD
Columbia University Medical Center
Department of Orthopedic Surgery
622 West 168th Street PH-11
New York, NY 10032
Tel: (212) 305-8188
Fax: (212) 305-4040
orthosrg@columbia.edu
http://nyp.org

New York University School of Medicine/ Hospital for Joint Diseases Program
Program Director: Orrin Sherman, MD
New York University Medical Center
530 First Avenue
New York, NY 10016
Tel: (212) 598-6509
Fax: (212) 263-8750
godetr01@med.nyu.edu
http://www.med.nyu.edu/orthosurgery

University at Buffalo Program
Program Director: Leslie J. Bisson, MD
University of Buffalo
Department of Family Medicine
462 Grider Street, CC102
Buffalo, NY 14215
Tel: (716) 898-5972
Fax: (716) 898-3164
psm4@buffalo.edu
http://www.ubsportsmed.buffalo.edu

University of Rochester Program
Program Director: Michael Maloney, MD
University of Rochester Medical Center
Department of Orthopaedics
601 Elmwood Avenue, Box 665
Rochester, NY 14642
Tel: (585) 275-5168
Fax: (585) 756-4721
karen_balta@urmc.rochester.edu
http://www.urmc.rochester.edu/ortho/ education

North Carolina

Duke University Hospital Program
Program Director: Dean C. Taylor, MD
Duke University Medical Center
Division of Orthopaedic Surgery
Durham, NC 27710
Tel: (919) 668-1894
Fax: (919) 681-6357
tinge007@mc.duke.edu
http://ortho.surgery.duke.edu

Wake Forest University School of Medicine Program
Program Director: David F. Martin, MD
Wake Forest University School of Medicine

Department of Orthopaedic Surgery
Medical Center Boulevard, #1070
Winston-Salem, NC 27157
Tel: (336) 716-3946
Fax: (336) 716-3861
hermance@wfubmc.edu
http://www.wfubmc.edu/School/ Department-of-Orthopaedic-Surgery. htm

Ohio

Cincinnati Sports Medicine and Orthopaedic Center Program
Program Director: Frank R. Noyes, MD
Cincinnati Sports Medicine and Orthopaedic Center
10663 Montgomery Road
Cincinnati, OH 45242
Tel: (513) 346-7292
Fax: (513) 792-3239
cfleckenstein@csmref.org
http://www.cincinnatisportsmed.com

Cleveland Clinic Foundation Program
Program Director: Mark S. Schickendantz, MD
Cleveland Clinic Foundation
9500 Euclid Avenue, A41
Cleveland, OH 44195
Tel: (216) 444-9507
Fax: (216) 444-7460
sportsfellowship@ccf.org
http://my.clevelandclinic.org

Mercy Hospital Anderson/University of Cincinnati College of Medicine Program
Program Director: Robert S. Heidt, MD
Wellington Orthopaedic and Sports Medicine
4701 Creek Rd, Suite 110
Cincinnati, OH 45242
Tel: (513) 554-8091
Fax: (513) 588-2484
rgwin@wellingtonortho.com
http://www.orthosurg.net/cincinnati- sports-fellowship

Ohio State University Hospital Program
Program Director: Christopher C.
    Kaeding, MD
The Ohio State University Sports
    Medicine Center
2050 Kenny Road, Pavilion Suite 3100
Columbus, OH 43221
Tel: (614) 293-8813
Fax: (614) 293-4399
amber.thompson2@osumc.edu
http://ortho.osu.edu

Pennsylvania

*Penn State University/Milton S. Hershey
    Medical Center Program*
Program Director: Wayne J. Sebastianelli,
    MD
Milton S. Hershey Medical Center
Department of Orthopaedics and
    Rehabilitation
30 Hope Drive, E.C.089
Hershey, PA 17033
Tel: (717) 531-4833
Fax: (717) 531-0498
jwoodley@hmc.psu.edu
http://www.pennstatehershey.org

*Pennsylvania Hospital of the University of
    Pennsylvania Health System Program*
Program Director: Arthur R. Bartolozzi,
    MD
Pennsylvania Hospital
800 Spruce Street
Philadelphia, PA 19107
Tel: (215) 829-2205
Fax: (215) 829-2478
valarie.dallas@uphs.upenn.edu
http://www.uphs.upenn.edu/ortho

Thomas Jefferson University Program
Program Director: Michael G. Ciccotti,
    MD
Thomas Jefferson University
Department of Orthopaedic Surgery
1015 Walnut Street, Room 801 Curtis
Philadelphia, PA 19107
Tel: (215) 955-1500
Fax: (215) 503-0530
susan.randolph@jefferson.edu
http://www.tjuhortho.org

*University of Pittsburgh Medical Center
    Medical Education Program*
Program Director: Christopher D.
    Harner, MD
UPMC Center for Sports Medicine
3200 South Water Street
Pittsburgh, PA 15203
Tel: (412) 432-3662
Fax: (412) 432-3690
dettyj@upmc.edu
http://www.orthonet.pitt.edu

Rhode Island

Brown University Program
Program Director: Paul D. Fadale, MD
University Orthopaedics, Inc
2 Dudley Street, Suite 200
Providence, RI 02905
Tel: (401) 457-1538
Fax: (401) 831-5926
scastle@universityorthopedics.com
http://biomed.brown.edu/orthopaedics

South Carolina

*Steadman Hawkins Clinic of the Carolinas
    Program*
Program Director: Richard J. Hawkins,
    MD
Steadman Hawkins Clinic of the
    Carolinas
200 Patewood Drive, Suite C 100
Greenville, SC 29615
Tel: (864) 585-4595
Fax: (864) 454-8265
cecilia.hanna@orfc.org
http://www.steadmanhawkinscc.com

Tennessee

*Sports, Orthopedics, and Spine Educational
    Foundation Program*
Program Director: Keith D. Nord, MD
Sports, Orthopedics, and Spine
    Educational Foundation
569 Skyline Drive, Suite 100
Jackson, TN 38301
Tel: (731) 427-7888
Fax: (731) 421-6597
http://www.sportsorthospine.com

University of Tennessee Program
Program Director: Frederick M. Azar, MD
Campbell Clinic-University of Tennessee
1211 Union Avenue, Suite 510
Memphis, TN 38104
Tel: (901) 759-3274
Fax: (901) 759-3278
rgraham5@utmem.edu
http://www.utmem.edu/ortho

Vanderbilt University Program
Program Director: John E. Kuhn, MD, MS
Vanderbilt Orthopaedic Institute
Medical Center East
1215 21st Avenue South
South Tower, Suite 4200
Nashville, TN 37232
Tel: (615) 322-9009
Fax: (615) 343-9073
colette.c.barrett@vanderbilt.edu
http://www.vanderbilthealth.com/orthopaedics

Texas

Baylor College of Medicine Program
Program Director: Walter R. Lowe, MD
Baylor College of Medicine
Department of Orthopedic Surgery
1709 Dryden Road, 12th Floor
Houston, TX 77030
Tel: (713) 986-7390
Fax: (713) 986-5591
ortho@bcm.edu
http://www.bcm.edu

Methodist Hospital (Houston) Program
Program Director: David Lintner, MD
Methodist Hospital (Houston)
6560 Fannin Street, #400
Houston, TX 77030
Tel: (713) 441-4879
Fax: (713) 790-1107
jmasterson@tmhs.org
http://www.methodisthealth.com

Plano Orthopedic and Sports Medicine Center Program
Program Director: F. Alan Barber, MD
Plano Orthopedic and Sports Medicine Center
5228 West Plano Parkway
Plano, TX 75093
Tel: (972) 250-5700
Fax: (972) 250-5747
khalligan@posmc.com
http://www.posmc.com

Texas Tech University (Lubbock) Program
Program Director: Richard Jon Pfeiffer, MD
Texas Tech University Health Sciences Center
3601 4th Street, MS 9436
Lubbock, TX 79430
Tel: (806) 743-2465
Fax: (806) 743-1305
somadm@ttuhsc.edu
http://www.ttuhsc.edu/som/Ortho

University of Texas Health Science Center at San Antonio/Nix Medical Center Program
Program Director: Jesse C. DeLee, MD
The San Antonio Orthopaedic Group
Santa Rosa Northwest, Tower 1
2829 Babcock Road, Suite 700
San Antonio, TX 78229
Tel: (210) 593-1477
Fax: (210) 804-5471
klawler@tsaog.com
http://www.tsaog.com

University of Texas at Houston Program
Program Director: Leland Winston, MD
University of Texas Medical School at Houston
Department of Orthopaedic Surgery
6410 Fannin Street, Suite 1535
Houston, TX 77030
Tel: (713) 799-2429
Fax: (713) 790-0505
kristey.tedder@uth.tmc.edu
http://www.uth.tmc.edu/ortho

Utah

University of Utah Program
Program Director: Robert T. Burks, MD
University of Utah Orthopaedic Center
590 Wakara Way
Salt Lake City, UT 84108
Tel: (801) 587-5455
Fax: (801) 581-5411
cynthia.murakami@hsc.utah.edu
http://medicine.utah.edu

Virginia

Orthopaedic Research of Virginia Program
Program Director: John F. Meyers, MD
Orthopaedic Research of Virginia
7660 East Parham Road, Suite 207
Richmond, VA 23294
Tel: (804) 527-5960
Fax: (804) 527-5961
fellowship@orv.com
http://www.orv.com

University of Virginia Program
Program Director: David Diduch, MD, MS
University of Virginia Health System
1215 Lee Street, PO Box 800159
Charlottesville, VA 22908
Tel: (434) 243-0274
Fax: (434) 243-0290
drd5c@virginia.edu
http://www.healthsystem.virginia.edu

Virginia Hospital Center/Georgetown University/The Nirschl Sports Medicine Foundation Program
Program Director: Robert P. Nirschl, MD, MS
Nirschl Orthopaedic Center for Sports Medicine and Joint Reconstruction
1715 N George Mason Drive, Suite 504
Arlington, VA 22205
Tel: (703) 525-5542 x206
Fax: (703) 522-2603
nirschlfellowship@yahoo.com
http://www.nirschl.com

Wisconsin

University of Wisconsin Program
Program Director: John F. Orwin, MD

University of Wisconsin Clinical Science Center
600 Highland Avenue, K4/751
Madison, WI 53792
Tel: (608) 263-0888
Fax: (608) 263-5631
richardson@ortho.wisc.edu
http://www.orthorehab.wisc.edu

ORTHOPEDIC SURGERY OF THE SPINE

Florida

Jackson Memorial Hospital/Jackson Health System Program
Program Director: Frank J. Eismont, MD
University of Miami, Leonard M. Miller School of Medicine
Department of Orthopaedics (D-27)
PO Box 016960
Miami, FL 33101
Tel: (305) 585-1315
Fax: (305) 324-7658
orthoapp@med.miami.edu
http://www.jhsmiami.org

Illinois

Rush University Medical Center Program
Program Director: Howard S. An, MD
Rush University Medical Center
1653 West Congress Parkway
Room 1471, Jelke Building
Chicago, IL 60612
Tel: (312) 942-5850
Fax: (312) 942-2101
beverly_kendall-morgan@rush.edu
http://www.rush.edu

Maryland

University of Maryland Program
Program Director: Steven Ludwig, MD
University of Maryland Medical Center
22 South Greene Street, S11B
Baltimore, MD 21201
Tel: (410) 448-6400
Fax: (410) 328-0534
cdickerson@umoa.umm.edu
http://www.umm.edu/orthopaedic

Massachusetts

Beth Israel Deaconess Medical Center/
Harvard Medical School Program
Program Director: Kevin J. McGuire,
MD, MS
Beth Israel Deaconess Medical Center
330 Brookline Avenue, Stoneman 10
Boston, MA 02215
Tel: (617) 667-2140
Fax: (617) 667-2155
selewis@bidmc.harvard.edu
http://www.bidmc.org

Michigan

William Beaumont Hospital Program
Program Director: Jeffrey S. Fischgrund,
MD
William Beaumont Hospital
3535 West Thirteen Mile Road, #744
Royal Oak, MI 48073
Tel: (248) 551-0426
Fax: (248) 551-5404
cmusich@beaumonthospitals.com
https://www.beaumonthospitals.com/gme

Minnesota

Twin Cities Spine Center Program
Program Director: Ensor E. Transfeldt,
MD
Twin Cities Spine Center, Piper Building
913 East 26th Street, Suite 600
Minneapolis, MN 55404
Tel: (612) 775-6257
Fax: (612) 775-6222
education@tcspine.com
http://www.tcspine.com

Missouri

Washington University/Barnes-Jewish
Hospital/St. Louis Children's Hospital
Consortium Program
Program Director: Keith H. Bridwell,
MD
Washington University School of
Medicine
660 S Euclid Avenue, Campus Box 8233
St. Louis, MO 63110
Tel: (314) 747-2536

Fax: (314) 747-2600
iffrigt@wudosis.wustl.edu
http://www.ortho.wustl.edu

New York

Hospital for Special Surgery/Cornell
Medical Center Program
Program Director: James Farmer, MD
Hospital for Special Surgery
535 East 70th Street
New York, NY 10021
Tel: (212) 606-1466
Fax: (212) 606-1477
academictraining@hss.edu
http://www.hss.edu

New York University School of Medicine/
Hospital for Joint Diseases Program
Program Director: Thomas J. Errico, MD
New York University Hospital for Joint
Diseases
301 East 17th Street, Room 1402
New York, NY 10003
Tel: (212) 598-6509
Fax: (212) 263-7180
randie.godette@nyumc.org
http://www.med.nyu.edu/hjd/hjdspine

SUNY Upstate Medical University Program
Program Director: Stephen A. Albanese,
MD
SUNY Upstate Medical University
4400 University Hospital
750 East Adams Street
Syracuse, NY 13210
Tel: (315) 464-5226
Fax: (315) 464-6470
bordeauj@upstate.edu
http://www.upstate.edu/ortho

Texas

Texas Back Institute Program
Program Director: Richard Guyer, MD
Texas Back Institute
6020 West Park Road, Suite 200
Plano, TX 75093
Tel: (972) 608-5148
Fax: (972) 608-5137
plane@texasback.com
http://www.texasback.com

Virginia

University of Virginia Program
Program Director: Francis Shen, MD
University of Virginia Health System
Department of Orthopaedic Surgery
PO Box 800159
Charlottesville, VA 22908
Tel: (434) 243-0291
Fax: (434) 243-0242
mcf3f@virginia.edu
http://www.healthsystem.virginia.edu

ORTHOPEDIC TRAUMA

Maryland

University of Maryland Program
Program Director: William C. Chiu, MD
University of Maryland Medical Center
22 South Greene Street, Room T3R32
Baltimore, MD 21201
Tel: (410) 328-3587
Fax: (410) 328-8925
sjordan@umm.edu
http://www.umm.edu

New Jersey

*UMDNJ-Cooper University Medical
    Center Program*
Program Director: Robert F. Ostrum, MD
Cooper University Hospital
3 Cooper Plaza, Suite 408
Camden, NJ 08103
Tel: (856) 342-3206
Fax: (856) 968-8288
ostrum-robert@cooperhealth.edu
http://www.cooperhealth.org

New Mexico

University of New Mexico Program
Program Director: Thomas A. DeCoster,
    MD
University of New Mexico School of
    Medicine
Department of Orthopaedics
1 University of New Mexico, MSC10
    5600
Albuquerque, NM 87131
Tel: (505) 272-6472

Fax: (505) 272-8098
jroberts@salud.unm.edu
http://hsc.unm.edu/som

New York

*Hospital for Special Surgery/Cornell
    Medical Center Program*
Program Director: David L. Helfet, MD
Hospital for Special Surgery
535 East 70th Street
New York, NY 10021
Tel: (212) 606-1888
Fax: (212) 628-4473
academictraining@hss.edu
http://www.hss.edu

North Carolina

Carolinas Medical Center Program
Program Director: James F. Kellam, MD
Carolinas Medical Center
Department of Orthopaedic Surgery
PO Box 32861
Charlotte, NC 28232
Tel: (704) 355-6046
Fax: (704) 355-7902
pat.hines@carolinashealthcare.org
http://www.carolinasmedicalcenter.org

Ohio

University of Toledo Program
Program Director: Nabil A. Ebraheim,
    MD
The University of Toledo Medical Center
Department of Orthopaedic Surgery
3065 Arlington Avenue
Dowling Hall, 2nd floor
Toledo, OH 43614
Tel: (419) 383-4020
Fax: (419) 383-3526
matthew.widmer@utoledo.edu
http://www.utoledo.edu/med/depts/
    ortho

Virginia

*Virginia Commonwealth University Health
    System Program*
Program Director: Mark C. Willis, MD
Virginia Commonwealth University,
    School of Medicine

Department of Orthopaedic Surgery
PO Box 980153
Richmond, VA 23298
Tel: (804) 827-1204
Fax: (804) 827-1728
orthoresprog@vcu.edu
http://www.orthopaedics.vcu.edu

PEDIATRIC ORTHOPEDICS

California

Orthopaedic Hospital/UCLA Program
Program Director: James V. Luck, MD
Orthopaedic Medical Center Campus
2400 South Flower Street
Los Angeles, CA 90007
Tel: (213) 742-1369
Fax: (213) 742-1435
nhamasak@laoh.ucla.edu
http://www.orthohospital.org

Delaware

*Alfred I. duPont Hospital for Children-
Nemours Program*
Program Director: William G.
Mackenzie, MD
Alfred I. duPont Hospital for Children
1600 Rockland Road
Wilmington, DE 19803
Tel: (302) 651-5890
Fax: (302) 651-5951
nmcox@nemours.org
http://www.nemours.org/hospital/de/
aidhc.html

Florida

Orlando Health Program
Program Director: Charles T. Price, MD
Orlando Regional Healthcare
86 West Underwood Street
Orlando, FL 32806
Tel: (321) 841-4499
Fax: (407) 650-7550
julie.brown@orlandohealth.org
http://www.orlandohealth.com

Georgia

*Children's Healthcare of Atlanta/Scottish
Rite Program*
Program Director: Raymond T. Morrissy,
MD
Children's Healthcare of Atlanta at
Scottish Rite
5445 Meridian Mark Road, Suite 250
Atlanta, GA 30342
Tel: (404) 255-1933
Fax: (678) 686-6866
mandy.rosenberg@choa.org
http://www.choa.org

Hawaii

*Shriners Hospitals for Children (Honolulu)
Program*
Program Director: Ellen M. Raney, MD
Shriners Hospitals for Children
1310 Punahou Street
Honolulu, HI 96826
Tel: (808) 951-3638
Fax: (808) 942-8573
ellen.raney@residentswap.org
http://www.shrinershq.org/Hospitals

Louisiana

*Louisiana State University/Children's
Hospital Program*
Program Director: Stephen D. Heinrich,
MD, MS
Children's Hospital
200 Henry Clay Avenue
New Orleans, LA 70118
Tel: (504) 896-9569
Fax: (504) 896-9849
sheinric@chnola.org
http://chnola.org

Massachusetts

Children's Hospital Boston Program
Program Director: James R. Kasser, MD
Children's Hospital Boston
300 Longwood Avenue
Boston, MA 02115
Tel: (857) 218-4924
Fax: (617) 730-0465
eliana.bolanos@childrens.harvard.edu
http://www.childrenshospital.org

Michigan

University of Michigan Program
Program Director: Frances A. Farley, MD
University of Michigan Health System
Department of Orthopaedic Surgery
(Pediatrics)
1500 East Medical Center Drive
2912 Taubman Center Drive, Box 5328
Ann Arbor, MI 48109
Tel: (734) 936-5694
Fax: (734) 615-8568
dzink@med.umich.edu
http://www.med.umich.edu/ortho

Minnesota

University of Minnesota Program
Program Director: Kevin Walker, MD
Gillette Children's Specialty Healthcare
200 University Avenue East
St. Paul, MN 55101
Tel: (651) 229-3948
Fax: (651) 312-3188
walke009@umn.edu
http://www.med.umn.edu/ortho

Missouri

*St. Louis Shriners Hospital/Children's
Pediatric Orthopaedic Program*
Program Director: Perry L. Schoenecker,
MD
2001 South Lindbergh Boulevard
St. Louis, MO 63131-3597
Tel: (314) 432-3600
Fax: (314) 872-7808
mturnipseed@shrinenet.org
http://www.shrinershq.org/Hospitals

New York

*Hospital for Special Surgery/Cornell
Medical Center Program*
Program Director: Roger Widmann, MD
Hospital for Special Surgery
535 East 70th Street
New York, NY 10021
Tel: (212) 606-1325
Fax: (212) 717-0673
academictraining@hss.edu
http://www.hss.edu

*New York University School of Medicine/
Hospital for Joint Diseases Program*
Program Director: Wallace B. Lehman,
MD
NYU Hospital for Joint Diseases
301 East 17th Street
New York, NY 10003
Tel: (212) 598-6509
Fax: (212) 598-6084
randie.godette@nyumc.org
http://www.med.nyu.edu/orthosurgery

Ohio

*Cincinnati Children's Hospital Medical
Center Program*
Program Director: A. Atiq Durrani, MD
Cincinnati Children's Hospital Medical
Center
Division of Pediatric Orthopaedic Surgery
3333 Burnet Avenue, MLC2017
Cincinnati, OH 45229
Tel: (513) 636-1383
Fax: (513) 636-3928
janis.messer@cchmc.org
http://www.cincinnatichildrens.org

*Nationwide Children's Hospital/Ohio State
University Program*
Program Director: Martin Torch, MD
Nationwide Children's Hospital
700 Children's Drive
Columbus, OH 43205
Tel: (614) 722-3393
Fax: (614) 722-3373
teaya.rough@nationwidechildrens.org
http://www.nationwidechildrens.org

Oregon

*Shriners Hospitals for Children (Portland)
Program*
Program Director: Michael D. Aiona,
MD
Shriners Hospitals for Children
3101 Southwest Sam Jackson Park Road
Portland, OR 97239
Tel: (503) 221-3486
Fax: (503) 221-3490
maiona@shrinenet.org
http://www.shrinershq.org/Hospitals/
Main

Pennsylvania

Children's Hospital of Philadelphia Program
Program Director: John P. Dormans, MD
The Children's Hospital of Philadelphia
34th Street & Civic Center Boulevard
Wood Building, 2nd Floor
Philadelphia, PA 19104
Tel: (215) 590-1527
Fax: (215) 590-1101
oshea@email.chop.edu
http://www.chop.edu

Rhode Island

Brown University Program
Program Director: Michael Ehrlich, MD
Rhode Island Hospital
Department of Orthopaedics
Coop Building, Room 170.36
593 Eddy Street
Providence, RI 02903
Tel: (401) 444-5895
Fax: (401) 444-6518
michael_ehrlich@brown.edu
http://biomed.brown.edu/orthopaedics

Tennessee

University of Tennessee Program
Program Director: James H. Beaty, MD
Campbell Clinic Foundation
1211 Union Avenue, Suite 510
Memphis, TN 38104
Tel: (901) 759-3274
Fax: (901) 759-3278
rgraham5@utmem.edu
http://www.utmem.edu

Texas

Baylor College of Medicine Program/
Shriners Hospital for Children-Houston
Program Director: Douglas A. Barnes,
MD
Baylor College of Medicine
Department of Orthopedic Surgery
1709 Dryden, 12th Floor
Houston, TX 77030
Tel: (713) 793-3776
Fax: (713) 793-3779
lbias@shrinenet.org
http://www.bcm.edu/ortho

Texas Scottish Rite Hospital for Children
Program
Program Director: John A. Herring, MD
Texas Scottish Rite Hospital for Children
2222 Welborn Street
Dallas, TX 75219
Tel: (214) 559-7556
Fax: (214) 559-7570
louise.hamilton@tsrh.org
http://www.tsrhc.org

Utah

University of Utah/Shriners Hospital for
Children-Salt Lake City Program
Program Director: James W. Roach, MD,
MBA
Shriners Hospital for Children
Fairfax Road and Virginia Street
Salt Lake City, UT 84103
Tel: (801) 536-3600
Fax: (801) 536-3868
jroach@shrinenet.org
http://medicine.utah.edu/orthopaedics

SHOULDER AND ELBOW

California

East Bay Shoulder Clinic Program
Program Director: Kirk L. Jensen, MD
12 Camino Encinas, Suite 10
PO Box 1298
Orinda, CA 94563
Tel: (925) 284-5300
Fax: (925) 900-4545
kjensen@eastbayshoulder.com
http://www.ases-assn.org/web/fellows/
Fellow_Jensen.html

San Francisco Shoulder, Elbow & Hand
Clinic Program
Program Director: Tom R. Norris, MD
San Francisco Shoulder, Elbow & Hand
Clinic
2351 Clay Street, Suite 510
San Francisco, CA 94115
Tel: (415) 392-3225
Fax: (415) 928-1035
trnorris@tomnorris.com
http://www.shoulderfellowship.org

Florida

The Florida Orthopaedic Institute Program
Program Director: Mark A. Frankle, MD
Florida Orthopaedic Institute
13020 Telecom Parkway North
Temple Terrace, FL 33637
Tel: (813) 978-9700
frankle@pol.net
http://www.floridaortho.com

University of Florida Program
Program Director: Thomas W. Wright,
   MD
University of Florida
Orthopaedics and Sports Medicine
   Institute
PO Box 112727
Gainesville, FL 32611
Tel: (352) 273-7375
Fax: (352) 273-7388
stewaml@ortho.ufl.edu
http://www.ortho.ufl.edu

Georgia

St. Francis Orthopaedic Institute Program
Program Director: George M.
   McCluskey, III, MD
St. Francis Orthopaedic Institute, St.
   Francis Shoulder Center
2300A Manchester Expressway, #A101A
Columbus, GA 31904
Tel: (706) 322-2462
Fax: (706) 320-3227
mccluskeyg@sfhga.com
http://www.sfhga.com

Maryland

Johns Hopkins University Program
Program Director: Steve A. Petersen,
   MD
The Johns Hopkins University
Division of Shoulder and Elbow Surgery
10753 Falls Road, Suite 305
Lutherville, MD 21093
Tel: (410) 583-2850
Fax: (410) 583-2855
jnaz1@jhmi.edu
http://www.hopkinsortho.org

Massachusetts

*Massachusetts General Hospital/Harvard
   Medical School Program*
Program Director: Laurence Higgins, MD
Massachusetts General Hospital
55 Fruit Street, YAW 3200, 3G
Boston, MA 02114
Tel: (617) 726-7300
Fax: (617) 724-3846
kdent@partners.org
http://www.bosshin.com

Michigan

William Beaumont Hospital Program
Program Director: J. Michael Wiater, MD
William Beaumont Hospital
3535 West Thirteen Mile Road, Suite 744
Royal Oak, MI 48073
Tel: (248) 551-0195
Fax: (248) 551-5504
lindsay.cooper@beaumonthospitals.com
https://www.beaumonthospitals.com

Minnesota

College of Medicine, Mayo Clinic Program
Program Director: Joaquin Sanchez-
   Sotelo, MD, PhD
Mayo School of Graduate Medical
   Education
Siebens 5, 200 First Street SW
Rochester, MN 55905
Tel: (507) 284-3316
Fax: (507) 266-4234
price.natalie@mayo.edu
http://www.mayo.edu

Missouri

*Washington University/Barnes-Jewish
   Hospital/Saint Louis Children's
   Hospital Consortium Program*
Program Director: Leesa M. Galatz, MD
Washington University
Department of Orthopedic Surgery
660 South Euclid Ave, Campus Box 8233
St. Louis, MO 63110
Tel: (314) 747-2534
Fax: (314) 514-3689
galatzl@msnotes.wustl.edu
http://www.ortho.wustl.edu

New York

Albert Einstein College of Medicine at Beth Israel Medical Center Program
Program Director: Frances Cuomo, MD
Beth Israel Medical Center
Phillips Ambulatory Care Center
10 Union Square East, Suite 3M
New York, NY 10003
Tel: (212) 844-6938
Fax: (212) 844-6983
fcuomo98@yahoo.com
http://www.einstein.yu.edu

Columbia University Medical Center Program
Program Director: William N. Levine, MD
Columbia University Medical Center
622 West 168th Street, PH11-Center
New York, NY 10032
Tel: (212) 305-5974
Fax: (212) 305-6193
orthosrg@columbia.edu
http://www.columbiaortho.org

Mount Sinai Medical Center Program
Program Director: Evan L. Flatow, MD
Mount Sinai Medical Center
5 East 98th St, Box 1188
New York, NY 10029
Tel: (212) 241-1621
Fax: (212) 241-9429
amanda.mercado@mountsinai.org
http://www.mountsinai.org

New York University School of Medicine/ Hospital for Joint Diseases Program
Program Director: Andrew S. Rokito, MD
NYU Hospital for Joint Diseases
301 East 17th Street, Suite 1402
New York, NY 10003
Tel: (212) 598-6509
Fax: (212) 598-6084
andrew.rokito@nyumc.org
http://www.med.nyu.edu/orthosurgery

Ohio

Cleveland Akron Shoulder & Elbow Program
Program Director: Reuben Gobezie, MD
Case Western Reserve University, School of Medicine
11100 Euclid Avenue, HH5043
Cleveland, OH 44106
Tel: (216) 844-3233
Fax: (216) 844-5907
ellengreenberger@uhhospitals.org
http://www.clevelandshoulder.com

Cleveland Clinic Foundation Program
Program Director: John J. Brems, MD
Cleveland Clinic Orthopaedics at Euclid Hospital
99 Northline Circle, Suite 100
Cleveland, Ohio 44119
Tel: (216) 692-7774
Fax: (216) 692-7802
bremsj@ccf.org
http://my.clevelandclinic.org

Pennsylvania

Thomas Jefferson University Program
Program Director: Matthew L. Ramsey, MD
Thomas Jefferson University
Department of Orthopaedic Surgery
1015 Walnut Street, Room 801, Curtis
Philadelphia, PA 19107
Tel: (215) 955-1500
Fax: (215) 503-0530
susan.randolph@jefferson.edu
http://www.tjuhortho.org

University of Pennsylvania Program
Program Director: David L. Glaser, MD
University of Pennsylvania School of Medicine
39th & Market Streets, 1 Cupp Pavilion
Philadelphia, PA 19104
Tel: (215) 349-8696
Fax: (215) 349-5128
david.glaser@uphs.upenn.edu
http://www.pennmedicine.org

Texas

Baylor University Medical Center/W.B. Carrell Memorial Clinic Program
Program Director: Sumant (Butch) Krishnan, MD
The W.B. Carrell Memorial Clinic
9301 N. Central Expressway, Suite 400
Dallas, TX 75231
Tel: (214) 220-2468
Fax: (214) 720-1982
klozano@wbcarrellclinic.com
http://www.wbcarrellclinic.com

The Foundation for Orthopaedic Athletic and Reconstructive Research Program
Program Director: Gary M. Gartsman, MD
The Foundation for Orthopaedic Athletic and Reconstructive Research
6410 Fannin Street, Suite 1535
Houston, TX 77030
Tel: (713) 799-2429
Fax: (713) 790-0505
michele@foarr.com
http://www.foarr.com

University of Texas San Antonio Medical Center Program
Program Director: Charles A. Rockwood Jr., MD
University of Texas Health Science Center at San Antonio
Department of Orthopaedics, MC 7774
7703 Floyd Curl Drive
San Antonio, TX 78229
Tel: (210) 567-4420
Fax: (210) 567-6962
rockwood@uthscsa.edu
http://som.uthscsa.edu

Washington

University of Washington Program
Program Director: Winston Warme, MD
University of Washington Medical Center
Department of Orthopedics and Sports Medicine
1959 Northeast Pacific Street, Room BB1015
Box 356500
Seattle, WA 98195
Tel: (206) 543-3690
Fax: (206) 685-3139
warmewj@u.washington.edu
http://www.orthop.washington.edu

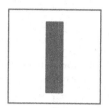

ABOS: RULES AND PROCEDURES FOR RESIDENCY EDUCATION PART I AND PART II EXAMINATIONS

A. Application dates and requests

1. The dates, locations, and application deadlines for Part I and Part II of the certifying examination are announced in the *Journal of Bone and Joint Surgery*. They are also listed on the Board's Web site (www.abos.org). Examination dates may be changed at the discretion of the Board. Confirmation of published examination dates can be obtained from the Board office.

2. To apply for either Part I or Part II of the certifying examination, go to the Board Web site and follow the directions from there. Printed applications are no longer available.

B. Application submission and deadlines

Part I. The postmark and electronic submission deadline for all required documents for application (those submitted electronically and those required to be mailed in) is **December 15th of the year before the examination.** These include:

1. Electronic submission of:
   o A completed application
   o A non-refundable application fee of $1040 online by credit card (Visa, MasterCard, American Express)

2. Paper submission to the Board office of:
   o The printed signature page
   o Other required documents (if applicable)

Both steps must be completed by the December 15th deadline.

Part II. The postmarked and electronic submission deadline for all required documents for application and case lists (those submitted electronically and those required to be mailed in) is **October 31st of the year preceding the examination.** These include:

1. Electronic submission of:
   o A completed application
   o A non-refundable application fee of $975 online by credit card (Visa, MasterCard, American Express)
   o A finalized, signed, and notarized original Scribe case list
2. Paper submission to the Board office of:
   o The printed signature page signed in 3 places
   o Signed and notarized hospital/surgery center letters
   o Finalized, signed, and notarized original 6-month case list from each hospital/surgery center

All steps must be completed by the October 31st deadline.

Late or incomplete applications and case lists. If the application and case lists are not submitted, or if any of the required documents are not postmarked by the deadline for Part I or Part II of the certifying examination, the application will not be accepted and the received documents will be returned.

1. If a Part I applicant wishes to submit the application and required documents by the late deadline of January 9th, the examination fee of $1040 and a non-refundable late fee of $350 must be submitted online.
2. If a Part II applicant wishes to submit the application and case lists and required documents by the late deadline of November 15th, the non-refundable application and credentialing fee of $975 and a non-refundable late fee of $350 must be included.

C. No applications or case lists will be accepted after the late deadline

1. When applying for either part of the certifying examination, an applicant requesting an accommodation in the administration of a certifying examination must submit their request along with documentation of the disability/need for the accommodation with their application by the application deadline. Documentation of prior accommodations for high stakes examinations should be included.

D. Notifying the Board of application changes

1. It is the responsibility of all applicants to notify the Board office of any change of address, practice association, or hospital affiliation.
2. If a Part II applicant changes practice location or practice association or acquires new hospital staff affiliations, new references will be solicited by the Board.
3. An applicant is also required to notify the Board of the denial of any request for hospital privileges; of any action to restrict, suspend, or terminate all or any portion of surgical staff privileges; of any request by a hospital to resign all or any portion of surgical staff privileges; and of any action by a governmental agency which would result in the restriction, suspension, or probation of the applicant's license or any right associated with the practice of medicine, including the entry into a non-disciplinary rehabilitation or diversionary program for chemical dependency whether by order or consent decree by the applicable medical licensing authority or on a voluntary basis.

E. Notifying the applicant of examination admission

1. For Part I, the applicant will receive examination information and a scheduling permit no later than 60 days prior to the examination date.
2. For Part II, the decision of the Credentials Committee is mailed to the applicant no later than 60 days prior to the examination date.

F. Fees

1. For Part I, the non-refundable examination fee of $1040 must be submitted with the application form online by credit card.
2. For Part II:
   o The non-refundable application and credentialing fee of $975 must be submitted online by credit card.
   o The candidate must also submit a non-refundable examination fee of $980 on or before the date specified in the letter of notification of admission to the examination. This fee will be forfeited if the candidate fails to appear for the examination or cancels after being scheduled.
3. The fees paid to the American Board of Orthopedic Surgery, Inc are not tax deductible as a charitable contribution, but may be deductible under some other provision of the Internal Revenue Service code.

FEES

Part I application fee	$1040
Part II application and credentialing fee	$975
Part II examination fee	$980
Late fee	$350

The Board accepts Visa, MasterCard, and American Express for payment of fees.

G Practice-based oral examination requirements

The Part II examination is practice-based. The purpose of the practice-based examination is to evaluate a candidate's own practice as broadly as possible. This exercise will be conducted much as rounds or conferences are during residency, with the candidate presenting his or her cases and responding to the examiners' questions and comments. *Applicants are urged to attend to details and follow procedures carefully and exactly in order to ensure admission to the examination.*

1. Case collection: Cases are collected in the Scribe program accessible through the ABOS Web site using the applicant's unique password and user ID. This case collection program must be used to compile the case list that is submitted to the Board. The applicant is to collect all operative cases, including same-day surgery, for which he or she was the responsible operating surgeon for six consecutive months beginning April 1 of the year before the Part II examination, provided that an applicant whose eligibility determination is deferred until the next year by the Credentials Committee may choose to submit a new case list or use the previously submitted case list unless otherwise directed by the Board. If time is taken off during the case collection period, the starting point for the collection period must be backed up by the amount of time missed. For example, case collection for an applicant who took a 2-week vacation in August would begin in mid-March.

All cases must be collected from each hospital and/or surgery center at which the applicant has operated during the 6-month period. If the applicant did no cases during the case collection period, this fact must be verified by a letter from the hospital and/or surgery center. The letter(s) must be sent to the Board office along with your case lists. This letter does not need to be notarized. It is understood, as stated in the practice requirements (IV, D) that the applicant during this period has been actively engaged in the practice of operative orthopedics surgery with independent decision making in matters of patient care. The case list must reflect this and must demonstrate ample cases to allow selection of material for the oral examination. A candidate must perform a minimum of 14 cases during the collection period to be considered operative.

Once all cases have been entered, the applicant will finalize and print the case lists by hospital. No changes can be made to the case lists after this is done. Each complete hospital list must then be certified by the director of medical records. The director of medical records' signature must then be notarized.

2. Case submission: By October 31st, the applicant must submit to the Board:

   o The finalized printed case list for the required 6-month period. Each hospital list must be stapled separately and have the required signatures and notarization. Before mailing, the applicant should make 3 copies of the complete case list(s) as the copies the applicant must bring to the examination must be of these printed and certified lists.

   o For each hospital or surgery center where no cases were performed, a letter stating that no cases were performed there during the 6-month period. This letter does not need to be notarized.

   This information must be sent to the Board office by registered mail or courier of your choice (ie, Federal Express, Express Mail, Certified Mail, etc) to:

   ABOS, Part II Exam
   400 Silver Cedar Court
   Chapel Hill, NC 27514

   Case lists must be postmarked by October 31st.

3. Case selection: The Board will select 12 cases from the applicant's 6-month case list(s). The list of 12 cases selected by the Board will be sent to the candidate in mid-April. From the list of 12, the applicant will then select 10 cases to bring to the examination for detailed presentation.

4. Exam materials/preparation: Once the candidate has received the list of the 12 cases selected by the Board, he or she must gather all of the following to bring to the examination:

   o Three copies of the list of 12 selected cases

   o Three copies of the case list summary sheet (sheet before the pie chart)

   o Three copies of the complication list

   o Three copies of the applicant's original, notarized case list that was submitted to the Board. The 10 cases selected by the candidate for presentation should be circled in red wherever they appear on the case lists

   o Three copies of notes and appropriate supporting documents for the 10 cases selected by the candidate. This includes admission and discharge notes, operative notes, operative consent forms, and office notes

- o Imaging (including x-rays) for the 10 cases selected by the candidate. The pertinent preoperative, intra- or immediate postoperative, and most recent follow-up x-rays for each case selected by the candidate for presentation. Before the examination begins, x-rays should be arranged in order of presentation and clearly marked in terms of date pre- and postoperative. Pertinent images in CT and MRI panels must also be marked. Any other imaging that is appropriate for presentation should be available for review during the examination

- o Video prints or photographic prints for the arthroscopy cases selected. The images should show the initial lesion(s) and the lesion(s) after treatment

- o For selected cases with complications, images (including x-rays) pertinent to the complication and its treatment and 3 copies of any consultation report(s)

- o Other materials that are necessary to support the decision making and treatment rendered

All materials for the examination must be in English.

All materials required to be brought to the examination, including all records, notes and images, should be organized and must be in their original form. Materials must not be altered or changed in any respect for presentation except as listed below:

1. Because the examination is to be anonymous, the candidate should remove his or her name from written material brought to the examination, including the 6-month case list(s), the complication sheet, the board's list of 12 selected cases, and the case list summary sheet.

2. To comply with the HIPAA Privacy Rule, candidates should limit the scope of identifiable patient information disclosed at the oral examination to the minimum necessary to conduct the examination. Therefore, you should **not remove** these items from the case materials you bring to present at the examination:

   - o Patient ID number
   - o Medical record number
   - o Patient name
   - o Patient birth date
   - o Medical device identifiers
   - o Serial numbers

   However, you **should remove** these items from the case materials you bring to present at the examination:

   - o Patient addresses
   - o Patient telephone numbers
   - o Patient fax numbers
   - o Patient e-mail addresses
   - o Patient Social Security numbers
   - o Health plan beneficiary numbers
   - o Biometric identifiers
   - o Full face photographs and comparable images
   - o Any other unique identifying characteristic

Failure to bring sufficient materials for the 10 selected cases to enable the examiners to evaluate the cases may result in the disqualification of the candidate, termination of his participation in the examination, or the withholding of scores.

Although the examiners will concentrate on cases brought for presentation, they may also ask questions pertaining to a candidate's case lists or practice. The candidate should not be concerned if all material brought to the examination is not covered. Discussion may focus on one area, or the candidate and examiners may become involved in a few cases in such detail that time will not allow presentation of all patients. In each examination session, between 2 and 4 cases will be presented to the examiners. The candidate will not be penalized for failing to complete discussion of all cases in their case list during this examination.

Candidates who have questions about materials required for the examination or the procedure for the practice-based oral portion of the Part II examination should call or write the Board office well before the exam. Failure to comply with the steps outlined may invalidate an examination.

Candidates are rated on the cases reviewed using this scale: 3-Excellent, 2-Satisfactory, 1-Marginal, 0-Unsatisfactory. Each case presented is rated on the skills outlined in the following table. The candidate's case list is also rated using this same scale.

CASE EVALUATIONS

	3—Excellent	2—Satisfactory	1—Marginal	0—Unsatisfactory
Data Gathering	Records all pertinent history. Records a complete physical examination. Uses imaging and other diagnostic studies appropriately. Records are complete and unique to the patient treated.	Records adequate history. Records an adequate physical examination. Adequate use of imaging and other diagnostic studies. Records are adequate and unique to the patient treated.	Records cursory history. Records an insufficient physical examination. Insufficient imaging and other diagnostic studies. Records are incomplete.	Records insufficient history. Records an inaccurate and/or insufficient physical examination. Unacceptable use of imaging and other diagnostic studies. Records are inaccurate and/or grossly deficient.
Diagnosis and Interpretive Skills	Synthesis of information gathered is complete. Formation of comprehensive differential diagnosis. Accurate integration of information to form the correct diagnosis.	Synthesis of information gathered is adequate. Formation of adequate differential diagnosis. Adequate integration of information to form the correct diagnosis.	Synthesis of information gathered is sometimes insufficient. Formation of differential diagnosis is incomplete, but not incorrect. Inadequate integration to form the correct and complete diagnosis.	Synthesis of information gathered is unacceptable. Formation of inaccurate differential diagnosis. Poor integration of information and/or formation of incorrect diagnosis.
Treatment Plan	Formation of appropriate non-surgical treatment plan. Formation of appropriate surgical treatment plan. Candidate obtains appropriate informed consent.	Formation of adequate non-surgical treatment plan. Formation of adequate surgical treatment plan. Candidate obtains adequate informed consent.	Formation of non-surgical treatment plan is incomplete. Formation of incomplete surgical treatment plan. Candidate obtains incomplete informed consent.	Formation of unacceptable non-surgical treatment plan. Formation of unacceptable surgical treatment plan. Candidate obtains inappropriate informed consent.
Technical Skill	Preoperative planning is comprehensive. Execution of the procedure is thorough and appropriate. Postoperative management is thorough and appropriate.	Preoperative planning is adequate. Execution of the procedure is adequate. Postoperative management is adequate.	Preoperative planning is incomplete, but what is presented is appropriate. Execution of the procedure is inadequate. Postoperative management is inadequate.	Preoperative planning is unacceptable. Execution of the procedure is unacceptable. Postoperative management is unacceptable.
Outcomes	Records appropriate patient satisfaction with care. Records appropriate objective measures of patient recovery at follow-up. Records appropriate attempt to maintain continuity of care.	Mostly records appropriate patient satisfaction with care. Mostly records appropriate objective measures of patient recovery at follow-up. Records adequate attempt to maintain continuity of care.	Records sub-optimal patient satisfaction with care. Records sub-optimal objective measures of patient recovery at follow-up. Continuity of care is incomplete.	Records unacceptable patient satisfaction with care. Records unacceptable objective measures of patient recovery at follow-up. Does not attempt to maintain continuity of care.

Case Evaluations continued

	3—Excellent	2—Satisfactory	1—Marginal	0—Unsatisfactory
Applied Knowledge	The candidate has appropriate knowledge of orthopedic conditions, diagnostic methods, treatment alternatives, outcomes, systems-based practice, and evidence-based medicine.	The candidate has generally adequate knowledge of orthopedic conditions, diagnostic methods, treatment alternatives, outcomes, systems-based practice, and evidence-based medicine.	The candidate has incomplete knowledge of orthopedic conditions, diagnostic methods, treatment alternatives, outcomes, systems-based practice, and evidence-based medicine.	The candidate has an unacceptable lack of knowledge concerning orthopedic conditions, diagnostic methods, treatment alternatives, outcomes, systems-based practice, and evidence-based medicine.
Surgical Indications	Appropriate, consistent use of accepted non-surgical treatment alternatives. The rationales for the procedures are appropriately described. Procedures chosen are consistently optimal and well supported.	Mostly uses accepted non-surgical treatment alternatives. The rationales for the procedures are usually appropriately described. Procedures chosen are generally well supported.	Inconsistent use of accepted non-surgical treatment alternatives. Insufficient rationale for some of the procedures described. Procedures chosen are sometimes sub-optimal or not well supported.	Inappropriate use of non-surgical treatment alternatives. The rationales for the procedures are poorly described. Procedures chosen are sub-optimal and unsupported.
Surgical Complications	Prompt identification of complications. Nature and frequency of the complications described expected for procedures described. Appropriate management of complications.	Usually identifies complications in a timely manner. Nature and frequency of the complications described mostly expected. Mostly appropriate management of complications described.	Identification of complications is delayed. Nature and frequency of the complications described are higher than expected. Sometimes sub-optimal management of complications.	Identification of complications is delayed or overlooked. Nature and frequency of the complications are severe and avoidable. Inappropriate management of complications.
Ethics and Professionalism	The candidate uniformly provides safe, ethical, compassionate, confidential, and professional care.	The candidate mostly provides safe, ethical, compassionate, confidential, and professional care.	The candidate inconsistently provides safe, ethical, compassionate, confidential, and professional care.	The candidate does not provide safe, ethical, compassionate, confidential, and professional care.

Financial Disclosures

Andrew E. Blustein, Esq has not disclosed any relevant financial relationships.

Dr. Kirk A. Campbell has no financial or proprietary interest in the materials presented herein.

Dr. Craig J. Della Valle has not disclosed any relevant financial relationships.

Lawrence B. Keller, CFP®, CLU, ChFC, RHU, LUTCF has not disclosed any relevant financial relationships.

Dr. Suezie Kim has not disclosed any relevant financial relationships.

Dr. Catherine Laible has not disclosed any relevant financial relationships.

Dr. Steve K. Lee has not disclosed any relevant financial relationships.

Dr. Daniel M. Lerman has no financial or proprietary interest in the materials presented herein.

Dr. Crispin C. Ong has no financial or proprietary interest in the materials presented herein.

Lava Y. Patel, BA has not disclosed any relevant financial relationships.

Dr. Carl Paulino has not disclosed any relevant financial relationships.

Dr. Afshin Eli Razi has not disclosed any relevant financial relationships.

Dr. David E. Ruchelsman has not disclosed any relevant financial relationships.

Dr. Eric J. Strauss has not disclosed any relevant financial relationships.

Dr. Brett Young has not disclosed any relevant financial relationships.

INDEX

Printed in the United States
by Baker & Taylor Publisher Services